Carolyn & Cancer
Some Days I Don't Feel Like Slaying Dragons

Carolyn Schreuer

Manor House

Library and Archives Canada Cataloguing in Publication

Schreuer, Carolyn, author
       Carolyn and cancer : some days I don't feel like slaying dragons
/ Carolyn Schreuer.

ISBN 978-1-897453-45-2 (pbk.)

       1. Schreuer, Carolyn--Health. 2. Breast--Cancer--Patients--
Ontario--Biography. 3. Teachers--Ontario--Biography.
4. Breast--
Cancer--Psychological aspects. I. Title.

RC280.B8S345 2014   362.196'994490092   C2014-906512-4

Cover design/realization Donovan Davie: 519-501-2375
Cover photograph courtesy the Schreuer family

Special thanks to Editors Lily Milanovich, John Paul Morrison, and Patricia Noel

First Edition. 192 pages. All rights reserved.
Published October 15, 2014
Manor House Publishing Inc.
www.manor-house.biz (905) 648-2193

We acknowledge the financial support of the Government of Canada through the Canada Book Fund (CBF) for this project.

Foreword

Every life has a beginning a middle and an end. This is the beautifully written story of a wonderful wife, mother, sister, daughter, teacher and friend to many people all over the world.

I was one of the lucky people to have shared my life with this awesome lady for over thirty years from a chance meeting in University to a peaceful passing in the Bob Kemp Hospice with just the two of us. Knowing Carolyn and how considerate she was to everyone she used her last reserve to make sure that happened.

Carolyn's gift to the world was her ability to observe and try and make the world a better place for those she encountered on her journey. One of her dreams was to be a published author and with this book we are fulfilling that dream and helping some other people along their journey.

This is Carolyn's story and her observations of the toughest part of her life. I'm sure her thoughts and advice will help many others facing difficult challenges of their own.

 Please enjoy it and by purchasing this book know you are helping people along their journey as well.

– Wayne Schreuer

This book is dedicated to:

My husband, Wayne,
my son Wes and
my daughter Victoria
who are my guiding lights,
the loves of my life,
and my inspiration!

Introduction

In April 2009, when I started on this journey, I had no idea what I was about to face. I had no idea about a lot of things and I thought I had my priorities in life, all straight. I had a great life – a great family, a wonderful husband, 2 great kids, a great job that I was very fortunate to love, 2 wonderful dogs that don't shed, a house I like, a swimming pool, air conditioning, and a cute VW car I like! I was mid forties, still pretty fit, and happy with my accomplishments and my life so far!

I was, back then, just completing my specialist qualifications for "Cooperative Education" through Queen's University! Taking this qualification would mean that I had more to offer in my teaching career and of course I know any extra education can never hurt! My goals were all becoming a reality. I was proud of myself!

My life was really coming along as I felt it should! I had great friends and a great extended family, a great social life and basically, I felt I had the world by the ass! I had arrived! My life was darn near perfect! Then - Breast Cancer?! Whoa! I didn't see that coming!

Never having had to face anything so scary in the past, I decided the best approach would be just to look it directly in the face and take it head on, one day at a time! I thought about who I would want to be, within the role of a "Breast Cancer Woman/Survivor" and truthfully, I suddenly had no idea!

All the accomplishments, all the things I had gained along the way meant nothing to me! What meant something to me, was my family, my friends and survival! Love & pain registered, but not much else.

After spending a great many years of my life striving to please others and still doing that to quite an extent, I told my husband right away, that those days were over.

From that point on, I decided to be completely real. I knew if I was going to face this, I would need all the resources that I could muster. I told Wayne that I was going to be real, and I would not be wasting any of my energy on manufacturing happiness to please others. I wouldn't be putting on a happy face if I was having a bad day! I needed him to accept this. I needed to accept what my emotions were and what I felt in any given moment and live through it. I knew I needed to respect my feelings as well as my body. That admission and philosophy came as a significant relief to me.

I seem to be crazed or blessed with an outlook that every cloud has a silver lining. Hopefully what I learned through this experience, can help me be a better person and live an even more productive, purpose filled, and valuable life. I hope I can share that with anyone who takes the time to read about my experience with breast cancer. It is my hope, if you find yourself faced with some daunting battle, that you too, will discover your own silver lining.

Here is my bent and twisted, sometimes unexpectedly humorous, brutally honest account of what I experienced during my breast cancer sabbatical. Life is all about the lessons! Experience really is the best teacher!

About The Title

Carolyn & Cancer: Some Days I Don't Feel Like Slaying Dragons

About 6-7 years ago before our good friend Joel Hall, was consumed and conquered by stomach cancer in January 2005, at age 42, we were out celebrating a birthday, having dinner with friends, and in a little book of signs that someone had given as a birthday gift, there was one in particular phrase, that stood out for me, and I adopted it as my own: Some days I don't feel like slaying dragons.

The phrase had a speckled place in my past, as an expression that appealed to me. Now, it works for me to describe the unwelcome battle that I was called to fight, and I am so grateful for the strength and courage I somehow found, even on those dark days when I needed to "slay the dragon".

Even before Breast Cancer, there were some days, I will admit, that I was not up for slaying the dragon. As a high school teacher, you always need to be tuned in, at the helm, commanding, and ready to stand up to defend virtue, or take action. We are all dragon slayers ~ you, me, and every one of my BC sisters who have fought this battle, and are still fighting.

Keeping this in mind, I hope what I have shared is a completely real account of what mattered during my Breast Cancer Sabbatical!

Contents

Foreword

1. In the Beginning

2. Tough Stuff

3. Pink Love

4. Tests and Other Freaky Stuff

5. Hope, Kindness and Inspiration

6. Hospital Culture

7. Chemotherapy

8. Radiation

9. Considering Reconstruction

10. Emotional Support

11. Self Esteem

12. Saving My Sanity

13. Respecting And Accepting My Body

14. Choosing Reconstruction

15. Finding a Lump

About The Author

1 In The Beginning

"Life is not a dress rehearsal!"
Monday, April 6, 2009

Somewhere in the back of my brain, there is a red light on and an alarm sounding – still quietly, but I know it's there. It's impossible to ignore.

Here it begins! It's a dismal, grey Monday and it's way too cold for April. What happened to that beautiful sunny day we had yesterday? Last night I kept waking up – which is so rare for me – hearing the freezing rain attack the windows, making a loud continuous smacking sound. I noticed 4am, then various minutes before & after 5am, then 6am and finally fell nicely back asleep when my 6:30 alarm with the radio mysteriously too loud, sent an adrenaline rush directly to my heart! It was like the scene on ER when they apply the paddles to the patient's chest & yell, "CLEAR!" My body jolted, but fell back down into place on the bed.

My 1ˢᵗ Mammogram
(Discovering the truth about my "little dill pickle")

This is not a typical Monday. I don't really mind Mondays. Today I had an appointment at the Henderson Hospital for my first mammogram. I'm 45. I knew I had a lump in my right breast. Over the past few weeks or so, I've affectionately named it "my little dill pickle". (I love cucumbers, love sweet gherkins, love fresh dill, but I've never been fond of dill pickles!) I was surprisingly calm about it all – shockingly calm and mentally together, way more than I ever imagined I would be… a little nervousness but remarkably together.   I drove myself to the Henderson Hospital and to go for my mammogram. I'm in the room waiting when I slowly begin to realize that I've got the hospital gown on backwards. I'm really no pro at this! I get 5 x-rays. (Squish X 5) Mammogram Guru Cathy is pleasant, and makes me feel as comfortable as one can feel while getting their boobs squished in a machine that groans. She handles my boobs like play dough, pushing them into place on the tray for squishing. I don't care and I am not the least bit embarrassed. It's medical and I need to find out about the pesky dill pickle that got stuck in my right boob!

I sit down in the waiting room, as I am told to do afterward, and try to read.   My eyes see the words but my brain is busy elsewhere. I command it back, and keep trying to re-focus. It's challenging! It takes me about 4 times as long to read an article about the philosophy of career planning and how it has changed, but at last I manage it and I think I remember what it was about. Then, I'm told I need to go back for another round with the boob squisher. Two more x-rays. Ouch, but it's quick at least. I can manage this. Cathy asks if I want to see the x-rays. Of course I do! She points out the masses that look like nasty, wild storm clouds in my right breast. There are at least 2 significant masses, that I can see, and perhaps even more. It really looks like quite a mess – and now, the dilemma - what will I call "it"?!   It's certainly no dill pickle!

Now for the Weather Report on those Storm Clouds

Cathy tells me I need to go for an ultrasound so I go back and wait & try to read again – this time a novel so big it hurts my forearm to hold it up for a long time, but I am determined to take my mind off the inevitable! I even manage to enjoy a chuckle or two in my novel, <u>The Secret Life of Edgar Sawtell</u> before I am called to ultrasound, across the hall. Dr. Blew, my family doctor, warned me about likely needing an ultrasound, so I'm not exceptionally nervous. I expect it. While waiting, a woman is in the changing room, trying to control her sobbing. I feel for her and a lump in my throat attempts to make its way up, but I force it back. I want to give her a hug, but I don't even know her. She probably just wants a hole in the floor to crawl into anyway. I continue to feign interest in my book, to respect her privacy, as much as I can, as I see that she is embarrassed and is keeping her head down, as she hurries out of the door. Ugh! That hurt... I felt her anguish as she swished by... I say a quick prayer for her.

Breast Ultrasound

"I'll have one ultrasound, 3 core biopsies, 9 loud clicking, boob smashing samples, and a sweet, girly martini with that please!" Yes, all on one bill...

Ultrasound Technician Amanda, is just back to work after tonsillitis, and still sounds quite sick.   Amy is her student assistant. Amanda is 35 and is hoping to have a baby soon. She was encouraged that my sister, who is 37, is expecting her first. Amy is in the Mohawk/McMaster program and has been hired there! She just got engaged and her boyfriend just got through testicular cancer. Lovely girls! They make me feel comfortable and are very congenial, which is a huge help because now I am starting to feel a little more nervous. I have the ultrasound. I appreciate the little things like the gel is warm, not cold. How thoughtful. Amy gives me towels for a pillow for my head and Amanda proceeds to hunt in all "quadrants" of my breast for more storm clouds. Sure enough, there is a real storm brewing there! She measures & charts the course of the storm and it takes at least half an hour – maybe more. She uses a black marker to draw on my breast to indicate where the "bad" spots are hiding. It's a little weird to have someone using a magic marker – I think it was a "sharpie", on my breast. It's nearly 11:00 am now and I've been here since 9:15.

Amanda tells me she knows they are going to want to biopsy the masses, which are "definitely not cysts". She asks me if I was planning to go back to work. "Yes, I am." I proudly & courageously announce! *(Of course I would go back to work. What do I know about illness or cancer or core biopsies?! I love my job, and besides, it is an excellent diversion! It makes me feel good!)* She asks what I do. I tell her I am a teacher and I am planning to do a promotional type of talk in a careers class at noon, to promote Co-op! *(One of my favourite things to do! I love the "sales" part, and it's such an amazing opportunity for the students. I feel enthused just thinking about it! I always do!)*

She suggests that I won't likely be feeling much like going back to work after the procedure. I have no idea how invasive this will be, but I take her word for it and call my colleague, Vesna to let her know I likely won't be back to work today. I want to sound strong because I know what Vesna is like and I don't want to alarm or worry her. I know she is thinking of me already. She is very concerned and offers to come & drive me home. How sweet! I assure her in my bravest voice, that I will be fine and if I'm not absolutely fine, I will promise to call her for help! I know if she comes to get me that I will turn into a big pile of sobbing mush. I can't let that happen! Not yet, anyway!

My Visit to Newfoundland

A sweet, female doctor named Connie Hapgood comes in to do the biopsies. She has a soft Newfoundland accent and I am immediately soothed by the sound of her sweet voice, and put more at ease. She has gentle, soft features; fair skin, dark hair but way too serious eyes. She's from St. John's and is only here for two and a half more months. She returns to Newfoundland in the end of June and she is looking forward to going home. I feel immediately comforted by her presence. I am grateful for that. Dr. Connie puts her hair in a ponytail, with the efficiency of a surgeon putting on gloves. I want to see the needle she is going to use. It's huge. I swallow and take a breath. I want to know how much they will take out. I have a lot of questions, but soon I am very quiet.

She freezes my breast & explains everything as she goes. I feel a little shaky but I practice breathing and my yoga concentration and it helps. Also the girls make conversation about Newfoundland, mountains & bears and the Rockies, weddings & honeymoons and my brain is able to transport there, if even only for a few moments, which helps too. I am in the woods from my childhood, hiking to the base of Gros Morne, the beautiful national park on the west coast of Newfoundland. I am 11 years old. I am sitting on a huge rock, taking a break, enjoying the breeze and the sunshine radiates on my freckled face. I am on top of the mountain, sitting in a patch of snow in July. I truly marvel at it all and feel so lucky to be privileged to feel so connected to nature and the planet. My dreams soar around me as I breathe in the wholesome air near the mountaintop! I feel exhilarated! I can see the breathtaking fiords on the backside of Gros Morne and briefly I am transported to a fascinating and carefree time and place. I am on top of the world! I soak it up and wish with all the fervor I can muster, I wasn't lying on the table having my breast turned into Swiss cheese!

Core Biopsies – *Get that Martini First!*

Then I feel the stinging, the pulling, the pressure and the tugging which seems to last forever in my stormy right breast. One mass is sitting on my chest wall, on top of my pectoral muscle. Hey, I never even knew about that one! I get two needles for freezing. Thankfully the pain is not bad but the pulling & tugging is giving me such a strange and uncomfortable, sensation. This is really,

13

really nasty. My brain suggests 'RUN!" but with a long needle in my boob, this would not be a pretty option. So I stay and endure... augh and it is particularly awful! I feel like the needle is poking through the underside of my nipple.

She takes 4 or 5 core samples and with each there is a loud snap and a little gadget squarely bashes me in the chest. Ouch! It's kind of like the ear piercing gun – startling, powerful and quick. Each sample biopsy seems to take forever and the tugging, pulling, pressure and discomfort continues. It's relentless! I tell my brain to go elsewhere and it reluctantly obeys for a bit. The pressure and tugging pull me back to reality. Ick! I think about a delicious, soothing martini that would have been so nice to have... The girls laughed when I asked if I could have one, before the procedure! I still think a martini would have been so nice! Thank God for anesthetic! It's my only true comfort at this moment.

The doctor takes 4 or 5 more core biopsy samples from the "storm" close to my chest wall. Then the procedure continues for the bumps on top, what I had formerly called my dill pickle. It's really horrible! Four or five core biopsies for that to get through – I lay there, as still as I can and endure, as women do. We endure. We survive!

Dr. Connie touches my shoulder reassuringly. She apologizes for hurting me and I tell her not to worry, I understand and I trust her. She called me Sweetie. I know she does not want me to hurt. I can tell. I can also tell that she is very concerned. She doesn't like what she sees. She knows. I know too. When the procedure is finished it's after 12 noon. It took a while. It was difficult. Dr. Connie tells me firmly and seriously, trying to give me hope, "You will get through this." I tell her I know I will.

Mostly I still feel mentally strong, but now that the procedure is over, I start to shake. Tears fill my eyes and the girls ask if I am okay. Amanda hands me some tissues and I tell them I think it is just hitting me. There is so much to take in and so much to think about. Surprisingly, my mind is not racing and I think I feel very coherent. No mental panic, which is what I would have expected. I know God gives you what you can handle! I wonder why this is happening to me. What am I supposed to learn from this?

A story is developing in my brain. Words are tumbling and swirling around me. I feel simultaneously afraid and calm. I felt like something entered me or perhaps my soul, perhaps it was an angel, but I did not feel alone. I felt a comforting, calming presence and I really felt the strength to face what lies ahead. I don't know how or why, but something changed in me that morning. I am grateful for it! I felt a transformation, a strength, and an intangible resilience, without any aggression. I can tell you if it lived within me before this morning, I honestly overlooked it. My perspectives are changing already.

Amanda wipes away some of the blood and applies an ice pack. I rest. Dr. Connie comes around to my front side of the bed and places her hand gently on my wrist. I tell her I am glad she is being honest with me. It doesn't feel too real at this point. It's kind of surreal. She asks me what questions I have. I say to her, it doesn't look good does it? I already know the answer. She gives me the knowing, attempt at a stoic nod of confirmation. I have to ask anyway. I have to say the word… I have to put it out there in the room, to deal with it. "Is it … cancer?" She tells me that the doctors read the biopsies on Mondays so we will get confirmation next week and then I will meet with my surgeon to discuss options. Dr. Connie pauses and then tells me gravely, with her words, "It is very suspicious." She tells me so much more with what she says with her body and her eyes. I know. She tells me that the surgeon will likely recommend a mastectomy, because of the multiple areas. I know it's cancer. I am numb. I think I am in shock. I think I am just dealing with it.

Dr. Connie holds my hand as I lay there on the bed and she looks deep into my eyes and she tells me, "When you meet with your surgeon, don't be surprised when he recommends mastectomy." Somehow, she is so reassuring, I accept this news as inevitable, already – a necessary journey. I don't know why or how I am accepting this. What is wrong with me? Why am I not screaming or angry or crying? It's like I already knew and Dr. Connie confirms my suspicions. God gives me what I can handle, I remind myself. Right now my breast is very sore and Amanda tells me when the freezing comes out it will be much worse. She cleans up more of the blood and then dresses the holes in my breast. We joke about it now looking like Swiss cheese! She tells me what to expect next - the pain, etc. but a fever or chills is a sign of infection and that should not be there unless there is a problem.

I ask Doctor Connie her name, just to be sure and she tells me. I don't want to forget her. Her presence was almost angelic. I felt strength from her. I'd like to see her again, but I know realistically, that it likely won't happen. She tells me, before leaving that she has seen young women like me who have gone through this and they are now in their 80's. I know she was giving me hope. Her reassuring words replay in my head, over and over again. Then she is gone.

Amanda tells me of some women who come in who have gone to Toronto after losing a breast to cancer and who have had reconstructive surgery. They take flesh off your tummy, do a tummy tuck and reconstruct a breast from the skin & tissue. They even make a nipple and apparently it looks very good. She tells me about some of the people she knows in the Juravinski Cancer Centre who are amazing people with great senses of humour. I know I will be getting to know them. I can tell. I make a few jokes and wish both girls well, and thank them.

I can't help but feel that they look at me like they wish I didn't have to go through what they know is inevitable. Thank goodness for the power and comfort of these women who have been my rocks to hold onto! Although we have only known each other a few hours now, they make me feel strong and reassured. I feel like I absorb strength and courage from them, even if only for a little while, but I am grateful. I thank God for bringing me this far, intact but I know soon I will be tossed in a tsunami of emotion. I feel so naïve. Maybe that is good – I don't know.

I exit the hospital in a semi robotic state. I find my way to the car on the rooftop of the parking garage. It hurts a bit to push doors open with my right arm, so I use the handicap door opener. It comes in handy at a time like this. I walk slowly, like someone who knows a tough battle is ahead. I am conserving energy – or perhaps it is that I have just been drained of energy. By the time I get up to the open rooftop where my car is, I can't be bothered to open up my umbrella. What is the point? Why should I care at this point if my hair gets messed up? How silly to be concerned about that. I almost scold myself.

I get to the car, take a deep breath and call my husband. I ask him how he is and then ask if he is "ready for a wild ride". I try to keep it together, but my voice caves and I can't hold back the enormous waves of fear any longer. We talk a bit and I tell him I am driving home. I wanted to be reassuring and not worry him, but he hears the truth in my wavering voice. Always a take charge and practical guy who does best when he can help in a concrete way, Wayne tells me that he will get some Tylenol for me and I will meet him at home.

Somehow I manage to drive home robotically, through the numbness and the waves of overwhelming emotion. When I get home he comes out to the car to meet me, which I appreciate. He has the Tylenol and has already started to boil the water to make me a cup of tea. How sweet! He hugs me tenderly in the garage.

He kisses my forehead. He assures me that he loves me and we will fight this. I so need to hear that! It helps!!! (Although many years before I have heard him say the same phrase about his Mom, before she passed away from cancer. "We will fight this...") I don't feel like I have any fight in me. I don't like fighting. I put that thought out of my mind.

On the way home, I drive without any sense of urgency. I decide I am going to write about this. That is what I will do! This will be my therapy. Raw. Honest. Released! Here it is.

My Story ~ *OMG! How did you ("THEY"!) discover "IT"?!*

Everyone asks the ever-burning question – and even if they don't ask it, you know they want to know. This is my story about how the breast cancer was discovered. Some time after New Years (2009), I noticed a small red dot that looked a little bit like a pimple on my right breast. This I thought was unusual, as I had never had a pimple on my breast before. I just thought it was odd and decided it was God's way of ensuring that I didn't ignore what was there. In January we had plans for a long weekend trip to Negril, Jamaica! We won the trip to Hedonism II and it was a dream we were really looking forward to – to say the least! I wondered if I had the nerve to enjoy a nude beach and I was looking forward to finding out! Also, I knew it would be a wonderful break for Wayne & I together! I had applied to take my 2 personal leave days off – the Thursday and the Friday just before January exams began and then we would have the weekend too. I noticed there was a small lump about 2 o'clock in my right breast but it was small and innocuous, so I thought. Because it was up high, it was easy to find and I could easily feel it when I was lying on my back in bed. I made a mental note to see the doctor about it, once we returned from our Jamaica trip.

January was super busy upon my return, getting everything finished up from semester one and getting read for semester 2. I got an appointment to see my doctor on Jan. 31, just before Semester 2 began. Unfortunately though, Dr. Blew was away that time, so I got to see her replacement, Dr. Mok – a 30-40 something female, her third day on the job, I think. I told Dr. Mok why I was there that I had a lump and a spot on my breast. She looked at the red spot near the lump and told me it was a "boil". I had no other symptoms, no fever just a little red heated area where the spot was. I'm 45. I had been feeling well otherwise – just a bit tired, but who the hell isn't tired these days?! Show me a Mom, or a working parent on the planet who is NOT a little bit tired. Good luck with that one! Not even worth mentioning that "symptom"!

No other questions. Dr. Mok casually told me, "Oh, it's just a boil – nothing to worry about. Take this prescription and if it doesn't go away come back in 10 days." I was not feeling reassured but I didn't want to question her professional opinion, or come across as disrespectful of her position. I did ask her once again, "What about this spot, this lump? (I insisted!) Can you feel it? I made her touch the lump and she again reassured me that it was only the underside of the boil – nothing to worry about. With that, I took the prescription and left, wanting to believe what she said, but not totally believing it. When I got back to my office, I told Vesna and she said, "You're not convinced it's nothing are you?" I said, no, but dutifully took the prescription anyway. Sure enough the red dot went away but the lump did not. What did happen though is that semester 2 started and life got super busy, with teaching all day and placing our kids in work place jobs, marking, etc. February was over before I knew it and Vesna & I were getting out to the workplaces to see how our students were doing at work! This is always a highlight of our jobs!

March was busy too! Wayne was launching his new business, Lockercity and we were all excited and anxious for things to get rolling. Suddenly it seemed, that I was in the ER with Victoria, the Monday night before the March Break. Around 10:30, she got out of bed to go to the bathroom and came over to our room to say goodnight to me again, as I was on the computer. She abruptly listed to the side and all but fell over with sudden, excruciating pain in her hip. She was unable to get herself back to bed! She couldn't put any weight on left her hip or leg and was crying and writhing in pain. We tried to console her with cold packs, & Advil and coaxing to sleep but it was clear that nothing was going to work! I called the nurse on call at Tele-Health Ontario and she instructed me to take Victoria to MAC ER right away, not allowing any weight bearing on the way.

Off I went to Mac, with my precious daughter in excruciating pain. It was the beginning of a long night and an even longer drama. We spent the whole night in the ER, not even getting past the door to Admitting until after 7am the next morning. We spent the next day there getting x-rays, pain killers, ultrasounds, and more x-rays unable to find anything. A couple of pediatric docs, grasping at straws wanted to give her a blood test. I knew that would do nothing but terrify her, which they succeeded in doing. I was not happy!!

Finally, before 4pm that day, Dr. Paul Missiuna came down to have a look. He took a brief look at Victoria's hip issue and said it's "greater trochanteric bursitis". He barely looked at her, but prescribed more pain killers and crutches and we finally got our ticket out of there! He also suggested physiotherapy, which we set up for later in March, once the pain was gone. Victoria was in complete agony all week and in additional to being horizontal, she was barely able to get around on the crutches. I took a couple of days off to be there for her as she couldn't even go to the bathroom or feed herself. I felt neglectful of my motherly duties and responsibilities and neglectful of my teacher duties too. It's always a very tough spot to be in. Victoria had to come first! By Friday evening of that week, she was beginning to be able to take a few steps with the crutches. We were elated and as the March Break progressed, it seemed she was doing better every day. I asked her is she was still taking her medicine as she told me what I wanted to hear – sadly, that was not the truth. By the Tuesday after the March Break, Victoria was right back in pain again and I felt like we hit ground zero all over again. I was angry at myself for believing in her when she told me that she took her medicine. I blamed myself for her pain again. Again, I took her back to see the Specialist and got more topical drugs and advice to help with the pain. Once again she was knocked horizontal for the rest of the week. We started physiotherapy toward the end of the week and finally Victoria seemed to be pain free – Thank God!

In the meantime, my tiny fingertip lump on my right breast had been changing. It was now more of an oval shape, which I light-heartedly nick named my "little dill pickle". As well, I noticed that there were some ways when I moved my arm in the shower that would cause my nipple to withdraw and pull in. I knew this was not a good sign.

With that, I picked up the phone to make the call I knew I could no longer wait for. I called my family doctor and asked for a mammogram. The receptionist put me though to the nurse practitioner, Mary, who informed me kindly but authoritatively, "We don't routinely give mammograms to women under 50." This was true – I was too young for a mammogram, but old enough to have breast cancer! Hmmm… makes sense right?!
I was not taking no for an answer at this point. Mary sensed it, and added, "You will need to come in first." After barely a breath, I said quickly, "OK, When can I come in then?!" Dr. Blew saw me on March 31 and my "little dill pickle" was now very easy to spot and feel and it measured on the outside approximately 3 centimeters across by 5 centimeters long. Not something you could overlook or call a boil, by any stretch of the imagination. Dr. Blew was very concerned and she got me in for my first mammogram as soon as she could, which turned out to be Monday, April 6, 2009. From this point, I knew I was in for a wild ride! I knew it was cancer.

21

2 Tough Stuff

April 7, 2009

I didn't sleep much last night.

I woke at 4am with a stiff neck and an aching breast. Oh, now it hurts, but I didn't feel any pain before the biopsy or the mammogram. Cancer came and threw a messy party in my breast and I didn't even feel any pain. It was so insidious! My mind started running and all it seemed I could think about is how people would be upset when they find out. Last night my Mom & Dad phoned from Florida and it seemed they had to tell me about everyone they knew who was diagnosed with cancer, dying with cancer or who has already died, from cancer. They're in their 70's so they know a lot of people who have died or are dying. Sadly, accounting for all these people and stages of misery is a daily pastime for my parents. They're not morbid or anything – it's just conversation – like a snowstorm or a change in the weather, or putting strawberries and walnuts on your Cheerios. I was quite proud of myself for keeping strong. It was easier than I thought it would be. I lied to them that everything was good and I didn't even have the slightest inclination to tell them otherwise. I had to lie. I knew I had to.

Back to work

Today I went back to work, which I love, and Vesna was there when I got in. I could tell as soon as we saw each other that she was going to cry. She gave me a big hug & had brought me in a beautiful bundle of home made cookies & treats that her Mom made! Lovely! We talked a bit and both started to cry again. Then we made a pact only to laugh. To start us off, I said, "Have I told you my right tit looks like Swiss cheese?" I said it looks like it went out to a party without me and had one hell of a time! We got laughing and that helped. Vesna got fresh water for the kettle and we made tea and caught up on what I missed yesterday and how life is going overall. I know she is there for me and boy I really appreciate her!

The day was very busy and it seemed like I was doing about 50 things at one time. It was a typical day, but now, I had an extra weight to carry and it was really weighing me down. Wouldn't you know, I had hall duty too, outside the Café. I wasn't very hungry at lunch time, but I forced myself to eat some broccoli soup. Vesna gave me some taziki and it tasted good! (Way better than the soup!) Cynthia stopped by while I was on Hall duty & gave me a little Lindt chocolate bunny, which I managed not to melt too much while holding it in my hand while I finished my shift of hall duty. I phoned Dr. Blew's office & left a message to ask if I needed to make an appointment for next week regarding the results of the biopsies. They phoned back later and told me no, they would get in touch with me and that I didn't need an appointment.

My breast and right side is still very uncomfortable and it causes me discomfort to move my right arm too much. I keep having phantom or flashback type of pains in the underside of my nipple. It's a horrible sensation. I feel very tender in that whole area. It looks nasty. It's bloody. Bruising has started and there are still some black marker lines. It feels worse. I keep popping Tylenol and have been feeling a bit nauseous too.

Wayne phoned me at lunch to see how I was & it was thoughtful. He phoned me again as I was just picking up Wes from vocal training. I was feeling very tired at that point. I just needed some down time. I just spent the previous 25 minutes or so, sitting in my car, waiting for Wes, holding my cell phone in case Victoria called. It's her very first babysitting job today so I wanted to be sure to be available for her. I dozed off a couple of times, but thankfully I didn't oversleep the 5pm finish time. Phew!

"Gentleness can only be expected from the strong. It is the weak who are cruel."

Oh, the helpful reassurance of others – *"Everything will be fine!"*

Wayne phoned me just as I was picking Wes up and told me that he told his brother Jim and Jim assured him that no one knows if something is malignant or benign, until they see it under a microscope. Jim works in the Hematology Lab in the Victoria General Hospital in Halifax and he has been a lab tech for over 30 years. Jim is a good soul and I know he was trying to be hopeful and helpful. I'm sure he wanted desperately to believe it's nothing and I know he would want to reassure Wayne.

I don't know why, but it irritated me that he knows nothing about what is happening to me, and nothing about what I endured or saw or experienced yesterday and yet he has to comment on what it might or might not be. Whatever... sometimes I hate when people try to console you with the old band-aid type of line – Oh, it's probably nothing... I know he was just trying to be helpful & supportive to his brother. I don't know why it bothered me. If he was looking at my chunks of boob flesh or my ultrasounds or the 7 x-rays I got squished for, then okay, give me your opinion, but otherwise shut up. It's none of your business. Don't tell me I'm fine. Don't tell my husband I'm fine. I don't like denial. I don't know why this bugged me so much. Nothing much has bugged me considering what I potentially have in front of me. My feelings surprised me. Of all people on the planet, Jim is an absolutely wonderful soul and I love him and admire him so much. He would do anything for anyone, and he certainly did not deserve my agitated thoughts! Hmmm... Why was this bugging me? I don't like it when people make me feel like I am over-reacting! Maybe that's why...

It was a long day really, even though it went very quickly – lots to do! Now I want to change our sheets and I desperately need a good hug and I need to finish the last assignment for this module of my course. I feel very tired. I feel like I could lay down now and sleep for hours! Only problem is that my lunch isn't made & I have a super busy day tomorrow and a very early start. I need to get there by 8am because of the Rob Ellis My Safe Work Meet & Greet & Assembly!

I think the emotional trauma; the waiting game & the pain are taking a toll on me.

Monday, April 13, 2009
Waiting...

Well, it's the end of Easter weekend and I am quite proud of myself. I actually managed to almost forget a few times, about the potential life changing news I will receive this week. My right side of my breast is still quite tender but the bruising is looking better. It's coming along and I can pretend that we might actually be able to resume our favourite playtime activities this coming weekend! What a happy thought. One day at a time, but now I am just really anxious to know – benign or not... I just need to deal with this. Perhaps once I know for sure, I will wish these days back – when hope is still alive... we will see... I guess no one really knows... although I do feel like I know. I do know... who is kidding who... I know it's cancer.

When I talked to Mom on the phone today, she mentioned about their friends who had just been visiting them and how their 30 something son who lives in Montreal needs heart surgery. Mom said, with disdain, well, finding that out really ruined their holiday! It makes me think that perhaps I shouldn't tell them anything until they are home and all is done, but it would be nice to have their moral support, I think. I don't want to be charged with ruining their holiday though. Now I'm not sure what is best. Something to think about… I better stop typing now as Wayne is in bed and I don't want to disturb him anymore. He is tired…

Back to work tomorrow…

Confirmation – *Yes, it's positive for ductal carcinoma*
April 14, 2009

Dr. Blew phoned me tonight when I was making dinner. I could tell by the sound of her voice that it was not good news. I appreciate that she is upfront & honest with me. I would rather deal with it than try to imagine what I don't know. The biopsy showed "grade 2 ductal carcinoma" and that needs to be removed. At this point she can't tell me if it has spread anywhere else except my right breast. Time will tell, I guess.

I will likely have an MRI and I don't know what else. She isn't sure of the treatments that will be recommended, but definitely surgery and perhaps radiation and/or chemotherapy. The surgeon will examine what is removed to see what it responds best to and that will be the recommendation.

Dr. Blew says that she will call me tomorrow with the appointment for the surgeon – either Dr. Ken Saunders at Henderson Hospital or Dr. Peter Lovericks at St. Joseph's Hospital. She says I could have the surgery as early as the end of this week or the beginning of next week. Suddenly it seems so urgent.

It's scary to think I might need surgery, so soon. Surgery! Yikes! The idea of surgery scares the jeepers out of me!

Wayne is having his final bowling night and he is looking forward to coming home & us chatting on the webcam – a first for us – but that is not going to happen. He will have no idea right now… I know he is hoping that all will be okay. I wish he was here so we could talk. I need a hug now and I have nervous butterflies in my stomach. Ick.

Dr. Blew says that they usually don't do mastectomies anymore but take the lump instead. I told her there were 3 lumps that I could see on the mammogram. She didn't know that. She said that it depends on what kind of cancer it is, etc. I think I'm kind of in shock but I want to just bury myself in my work – my course work. I'm swaying between numb & distraught…

I'm trying to be calm & just re-focus… I will be glad when Wayne is home so I can talk to him! I need some moral support. I hope he is up for this. I hate to have to give him bad news, but I need his support. I hope he can cope with this and what lies ahead for us.

Sunday, April 19, 2009

Well it's hard to believe I've been through nearly 2 weeks since the mammogram, and all that nasty stuff… and I knew what was coming… I knew it was cancer.

The days have been going fast but some of the nights have been going slowly & not because I have been sleeping but for the first time, I am waking up. It seems if I wake up at 4 or 5am, then I won't fall back to sleep right away.

Last night some noisy teens were outside the front of our house around 3:30am and they were yelling and making tons of noise getting cabs… I was awake for nearly 2 hours after that, and thankfully I didn't have to get up to go to work today. I used to always fall asleep before, without any trouble at all. Now I can't seem to be able to do that at all! I don't like that!

When I least expect it, out of nowhere, I get a punch in the gut!

It's strange how I can feel so normal & carefree at times & then suddenly, when I least expect things to crumble, I feel like I get punched in the face.

Friday was my toughest day yet. I went to see my first student and felt mentally, completely scatterbrained. I pulled out the wrong file for the student & I didn't even realize it. I gave the supervisor another copy of a report she had already filled out because it wasn't in the file – wrong file – why would it be there. I was hopeless when I tried to concentrate and I just couldn't get it together. It was horrible. I kept it together pretty much until I got to the car and then I was so disappointed with myself, that I just wanted to cry... I was so disappointed in myself. I phoned Wayne & left a message.

I pulled myself together a bit & went to see my next student. When I went to take a picture of Ashley, & her supervisor and the kids in the daycare, as they were all lined up, I frantically searched for my camera. I couldn't find it anywhere & I had NO idea where it could have been! I had to take a picture of the children with my pretend camera. They were good with that!

Later I thankfully found it in my trunk where it had obviously fallen out of my briefcase. What a relief. I had missed Wayne's call so I called him back & he was meeting with Dr. Blew. I was glad they were talking. I feel so glad I have Wayne to handle some things, when I feel overwhelmed. After my first 2 appointments, I felt like a complete idiot! I was so disappointed with myself that I just wanted to cry. In those moments, I couldn't focus if my life depended on it. It scared me. I'm usually so together & efficient. I hated that feeling.

Wayne got Ron Foxcroft on the case and he got me moved up to the top of the cancellation list – I think. I called in his chips & worked his network and hopefully it will be over sooner. I'm embarrassed at someone pulling strings for me because I am not any more important than everyone else in the queue. I feel embarrassed, but grateful, for sure!

It's so hard to tell the people you love!

The other thing that I have been finding mentally & emotionally exhausting is telling people I have breast cancer. I didn't want to keep the kids in the dark so we told them on Wednesday night. Victoria cried for hours & hours.

She woke up the next morning and still cried. Victoria made me promise that I wouldn't die. I promised her I wouldn't – at least not for another 50 or so years! Wes told me she cried a lot in school that day too. Wes was teary eyed but mostly he asked questions. Wes searched the survival rate on the Internet and informed me that most people survive. Wayne made a joke about all three of them having enjoyed my boobs. We laughed. Victoria still cried. I felt like her little heart was breaking.

Wes changed his Facebook status to being confused, concerned & worried. He sent text messages to his friends. He told me he was going to put my name in the special intentions for prayers box in his classroom & asked if that would be okay. When he went to put my name in, he found that his classmate, Victoria, had already done it. Portia, another girl in his class asked Wes to tell me that she hopes I feel better. Seems like the girls in his class were being supportive. I thought that was sweet of the girls to rally together in support.

"The angry people are those who are most afraid."

Telling people & Everyone Reacts Differently

I felt so nervous telling Randy, our Principal. He was very good about it and said he would do whatever I wanted him to do, to help in any way. He asked me a lot more questions than I expected, but I didn't mind answering them at all. (How did I discover it? When? What happened? Etc.) He was very sympathetic and supportive and he gave me a big hug. It's the softest side I've ever seen of him yet. I told him I might be off for 2, or maybe even 3 weeks! I figured I could be back maybe by the first week of June. There is so much that is unknown. I reminded him how not anyone can cover for coop, and I suggested that Steve Sloan would do a great job, if it could be arranged and if Steve was interested. Randy said, that he understood that I was concerned about that, but that really it should be the least of my worries. I told Cynthia the next day. She was shocked, supportive too. She told me that it helped her readjust her priorities. I was grateful something good came out of something like this!

I was dreading telling my parents and my brothers and sister. My Mom started to cry but I was able to remain strong and positive. I sure hope I can keep up this strength. I felt relieved and exhausted after telling them. My Mom seemed to take it hard. I consoled both of them as best I could, but I was proud that my voice didn't waver, so I think that helped them.

Marilyn called me back first. She had some questions & was concerned. I wished I could have had happy news. The good news was that the baby is kicking her all the time now! She offered my some of her FF cups for when the time was right. Generous!

Claudine was home so I told her. She was nursing Ellie from the flu as she had been up vomiting since around 1am! Poor Claudine! I asked her to tell Greg & then have him call if he wanted to, when he got home from work. Greg phoned a little later & I was out with the dogs. I phoned him back. The first thing he said after my "Hi! How are you?" was something inaudible, because of his tears. He passed the phone to Claudine. I said, "Claudine, tell Greg to stop being such a wuss & get back on the phone." We talked the longest and he told me about getting a core biopsy done on his leg last year. Little bugger didn't tell me about that before! It all turned out okay, thank goodness! Greg was the most sympathetic.

When Jeff phoned me back, he was kind of slurring his words and I couldn't make out everything he said the first time. He does this sometimes. He was all "Mr. Casual". Oh, everything will be fine & it's easy to fix and lots of people get it and it's no problem... and blah, blah, blah... but that's Jeff – Mr. Happy Go Lucky! Perhaps that is his way of dealing with it, but for me, it was the least helpful and it made me feel the worst. I know Jeff is a complete softie underneath that let it all slide off me exterior, so I know it hurt him a lot to hear what I had to say, and I know he didn't mean to make me feel that way. Everyone has his or her own way of coping but one way does not work for everyone! Denial does not work for me at all! Greg has always been the best communicator and we have always been the most similar, and simpatico.

I've come to realize that not only does everyone deal with this in different ways, but I find it helps me to have to comfort others and I am less comfortable with others making light of what I am dealing with, or what I am about to deal with... I think I am better at comforting than being comforted, unless it is by Wayne. Then I like to be comforted and protected and feel safe and secure.

Wesley sent me a text message and he said "I'm so sorry about ur cancer". I thought that was cool. After school he said to me, "I don't know how to react. Am I supposed to be afraid?" We talked a bit. He has been very willing to come on a walk with me, which I really like. Also, Wayne has been very willing to come with me to walk the dogs lately and I love that! It's a good chance to talk and reflect. Wayne has been so supportive and good. I treasure him more than ever!

Friday, after all the mental chaos I was feeling, I planned to leave work after lunch, as I had a hall duty. I tidied things up and handled a few things, emails, messages, etc. and planned to mark posters, but never got to that. I told Steve Sloan what was going on & I asked how he felt about possibly covering for me when I'm off. He was keen and willing to do it, which was definitely what I had hoped for, as I trust him & it would be the easiest transition and smoothest transition for Vesna.

Vesna called to check on me too.

Wayne called a few times to keep telling me to go home & chill. I ended up leaving around quarter to 2:00. My head was pounding and I was fried. I was asleep by 3:30 and Victoria woke me up around 7pm to have dinner, which Wayne made. It was so good & I felt so much better and so loved and taken care of. It was so good to be home. Wes brought me a "Get Well" card and a gift! He gave me the comedy DVD "House Bunny" and an adorable frog outdoor garden hanging ornament, a large Kit Kat bar and a Mars bar. I thought that was so thoughtful of him. He wrote in the card, "Dear Mommy, I love you and Thanks for being so strong." I was really touched by his thoughtfulness and his words! I guess there is another thing good coming from something horrible. Wes is maturing and thinking of someone other than himself.

Saturday when I went out with Victoria to buy a few things for Alexander's little welcome basket, I enjoyed the sauntering. It just was not in my realm to hurry around. I couldn't do it – even if I had to. I was going to run a few more errands but found I was too tired to bother & I was actually glad to be home on a Saturday night for a change. That is the biggest thing I find. I can't go as hard as I usually push myself. I think I will have to be more respectful of my limitations now and not burn myself out. I need to do some work on my course but I also felt I wanted to write more about the experience so far.

Still, the hard thing is to tell people. I like it when Wayne tells them for me. It saves me the stress. I feel I need to downplay it and then work to make sure the news hasn't brought them down. I feel it's important for me to leave them feeling cheered up, rather than upset. I try to help do this, but it isn't always easy!

Waiting

Also in the days that followed surgery, was the waiting… I was sure the cancer had been removed from my chest. My breast was gone to prove it. However, I wondered if it had managed to desecrate another part of my body before we got to evict this rude partier from my body. I wanted to know what next, what about the pathology? Were the margins clear? What happened to my boob? I thought of someone getting it on a platter in some lab somewhere, having the daunting task of slicing and quantifying all the findings. It seemed weird when I pictured my boob, like a little mound of Jello, nipple on top, jiggling on a silver platter, ready for dissection, or perhaps a squirt of whipped cream instead. Now that would be more to my liking!

What I didn't realize until later was that this waiting game was particularly hard on my husband. I just naively assumed that wherever the cancer was, that the chemo would eradicate it from my body. I call it blind faith in medicine and the doctors, but I

33

had every confidence that they would take care of me and that I would be cured. I would win. When the oncologist started to give me the statistics later, they went in one ear and out the other. I told my husband that statistics don't apply to me, because God gave me the determination of 5 people. This is something I have always believed and am grateful for! It wasn't because I thought I was super human. Looking back it was completely naïve of me to think this way.

Wayne, having lost both of his parents to cancer, knew that if the cancer had already spread to a vital organ then he was in serious danger of losing me. At the time, I had no idea how close I was to that reality. Three weeks went by and I was still waiting for the pathology report. I was wondering, what have they done with that old cancer boob? I hope someone is testing it and figuring out my "plan of attack"! Hmmm... Maybe they just tossed it in biological waste and they will just make something up! Finally around 3 weeks after my surgery, my pathology report came back and I got to learn the details of my cancer.

Just when I thought things would all come together and we would know our plan of attack, things fell apart for me emotionally. My family doctor was leaving for 3 months to travel with her family for the summer. My surgeon was going on vacation, so he couldn't translate the pathology report into plain English, and Wayne was going to be away. All my supports fell down around me and I felt the walls cave in on top of me. I needed someone to lean on, but today was not the day. It was the first of a few "down days" I would experience.

Telling the Kids

My daughter was 11 when I was diagnosed and my son was 13. The biggest thing we found critical, is not to delay telling them. They know something is wrong. I was planning on waiting until I knew the surgery date, but the atmosphere was too tense and they knew we were upset. We called a family meeting and both kids thought *they* were in trouble. They were wondering what they had done. I wish I didn't wait because they were upset that we didn't tell them right away. My daughter cried. My son got angry & went to the Internet to research survival rates. It was very hard on them, because they wondered if I would die. They were scared about me having to go to the hospital and have surgery.

There were a lot of questions, so I was very honest and forthcoming with information and feelings. They really wanted to be kept in the loop! It made them feel respected and they felt like they were an important part of what we were all dealing with. They were not happy if they felt like they were the last to find out anything, even if it was just an appointment date. I also took both children separately to a Counselor and we talked.

My daughter was internalizing a lot of emotion. My Counselor suggested that she write her feelings in a journal. She also suggested that she write down whatever questions she had too, so we could get answers. It was tough to see my children hurting. I wanted to comfort them but I refused to be dishonest and feed they any false hope.

I was brutally honest. It was tough. But we got through it. I think the best thing is to give them permission to ask questions and it's okay to feel whatever they feel. It's so important to keep talking, as much as they want to talk about it. It was also important to make sure they were heard and to ensure that we really listened to them.

What was hard for me:

The hardest part for me was feeling like I was letting down the people I love. It was also so hard to feel dependant on people and feel like I was a pain for others to take care of. It was hard to be a patient. I hate the feeling of inconveniencing people.

It's hard to think about the possibility of leaving my family behind, when they might still need me. If cancer comes back and takes me, I hope I can at least be here for my children when they get married and when they have babies of their own.

I do hope to be a Grandma some day and I do hope to be able to take my little grandchildren to the park and push them on a swing and catch them at the bottom of the slide! I do hope to be able to bake cookies with them, and eat the cookie dough like we always did with my Mom and like I do with my children now! Who will love and care about my children like I do?

It's hard to think that some day, Wayne might be left alone and feeling lonely! Who will take care of the silly things I take care of for him? Who will love him and understand him and accept him, like I do?

It was hard for me to express my gratitude to everyone who deserves so many "Thank yous"! I know I will never be able to write all those thank you notes, but I hope people realize that and know how much I appreciate their kindness!

3 Pink Love

One of the crazy things about having cancer is that people are suddenly motivated and willing to show you their love and gratitude! Lucky me! Honestly, there were a few people at work who I thought never really gave me a second though. I'm sure they didn't hate me or anything, but to think that they cared about me beyond a simple hello, was a stretch! Perhaps people suddenly think, "OMG, she has cancer and she is going to die soon. Maybe I should reach down deep and pull out something nice and kind to tell her, in case she croaks before I get the chance to tell her." Maybe it's not like this at all and this is another creation of my overly active imagination! Well, we will never know now, will we?! Here are some of the beautiful & wonderful things people said to me, or wrote to me, which picked me up and genuinely helped me through the day!

Wayne's sister Michelle wrote me an awesome email! She hardly ever writes, so when she does I always feel she has something important to say and I listen. On 16-Apr-09, at 1:24 PM, Michelle Schreuer wrote:

Carolyn,

OK - you are a strong hot mama who can control the world of several hundred teenagers, two kids and my brother. YOU CAN KICK THIS STUPID DISEASE IN THE ASS!

We love you. We know you can whup this.

Love,
Michelle

"You are one of my favourite people on the planet!" - Craig

Food, Glorious Food

The days that followed my mastectomy surgery, leading up to my chemotherapy treatments, were both difficult and glorious! My home turned into a fragrant flower garden as friends, colleagues and acquaintances lavished our family with an outpouring of love! I received some of the most gorgeous flowers I had ever seen. I was feeling liberated, knowing that the cancer had been cut from my chest, and even though it took my breast, at least it didn't take my life and for that I was grateful. The flowers kept coming! I was truly overwhelmed with cards, notes, fruit baskets, books, treats of all sorts, and shared feelings of compassion! People came out of the woodwork to do kind things for us and we felt so blessed!

Friends from our old neighbourhood in Stoney Creek showed up too, and one of the many gifts of kindness that meant a lot to us was the gift of food! One day I found a home made casserole dish of cheese tortellini, on our doorstep, another day, delicious lentil soup, banana bread still warm from the oven, banana & chocolate chip muffins with flax seed, salsa dip, vege lasagna and peanut butter balls for dessert! One friend, Marylynn, wanted to set the table for us, but missed us so she left in a box, a lovely silk table cloth, cloth napkins with gorgeous diamond napkin rings, elegant candles in holders, salad, bread, and dinner. Another friend showed up one day and brought lunch – everything I love – albacore tuna sandwich, complete with even green leaves candy for dessert. Some brought healthy snacks, decadent treats, cakes, brownies and gourmet cupcakes and home baked treats, fresh fruit and chocolate. Every gift was welcomed and consumed with delight, if not by me, certainly by my family. There were times when I could not stand the taste of anything and times when mouth ulcers from chemo left me completely turned off of food, but there was something about the comfort of food that people brought, that made us all feel loved.

Having an Atlantic Canadian background, I grew up in a home where we ate to live. We never lived to eat. I used to think of what to make for dinner by weighing in my mind, what would make the least amount of mess. My friend Lisa, who has Polish background, taught me a new philosophy, that "Food is LOVE"! I really wanted to embrace that philosophy! I can honestly say that the food gifts we received, definitely made us feel loved.

In those days after my mastectomy, before I lost my hair, and my appetite for life, when I was regaining my strength, while Spring was blooming, I felt a brief but powerful rebirth. Just being able to get outside in the sunshine felt so incredible. Feeling the sun on my skin warmed me to the bone, and I felt a new appreciation of life – all life – like something wonderful was growing inside me, only this time it wasn't a baby. I was experiencing things in a whole new way, seeing the world in a whole new light with a renewed appreciate for all the little things I had previously taken for granted. I remember walking with my daughter, holding her hand as we strolled slowly around our neighbourhood. Victoria didn't even care that I had drains coming from my body. She was 11. She was happy that we could just walk together, hold hands and feel the Spring sunshine on our faces. It was on one of those blissful little walks that the following ideas came to mind, "Great things about having Breast Cancer". (That list of great things will be coming up, so yes, you need to keep reading!) Well I guess you cold skim. I'll admit I do that sometimes. You'll never know what you will miss out on though if you do skim! It could be a steamy sex scene or some other titillating piece that you would not want to miss. Just saying…) I truly felt glad to be alive!

Flowers & Fruit Baskets and Cards – Oh my!

Upon death, I fed the green bin with those once beautiful flowers who had lived their lives, committed to the service of my pleasure! Those arrangements showed such radiant beauty, and now the drooping flowers were so ugly and smelly in death. So sad! So diminished. I felt guilty for all the lavish attention and the extravagant bouquets and wondered if I had reacted so graciously and thoughtfully when my friends were in need! I also felt guilty for all the money people had spent, just to send me flowers that gave me such pleasure, but were so temporary. I often thought about how I would have loved to know that hungry children were being fed instead of me getting to enjoy another bouquet of gorgeous flowers!

My Mom always used to say to us, "It's never too soon to be kind to someone, because you never know how soon could be too late." (Joanne Snow-my Mom)

Our 19th Wedding Anniversary ~ July 7, 2009

Today is our 19th wedding anniversary! I feel happier today and physically better, despite the aching in my left chest from where the port-a-cath (power port) was "installed" on Friday, July 3 – Wesley's 14th birthday. "Installed" sounds like a car part, but it sure wasn't that easy! Since no one has been here to change my dressings, I just got fed up and took them off myself! A little air will be good, I think. It's cooler today. So unlike July, normally. I should take the dogs out but each step hurts my chest where the port is. My sports bra strap irritates it. My gums are achy and my neck is very sore, but in terms of my intestines, they feel the best they have felt since my first chemo. So that is a real treat! Phew! Today I will see Dr. Arnold & Dr. Wadell (now Dr. Decarolis) again. I will also get more blood work done to see if my white cells are rising to the occasion. I hope so!

I do worry about our relationship. My hair is thinning. I have a port stuck inside my healthy chest side. It's ouchy. No position is comfortable. Even though I feel the tingling urges for sex, how can we possibly get into it? Somewhere is always ouchy. Wayne does not want to hurt me. He is being very protective of me. He looks at me like I have become fragile, and perhaps I have. Soon I will be bald as well. My mouth has sore spots inside – another side effect from the chemo drugs. Oh yes, I'm a beauty! A regular sex kitty! A real trip to Hollywood! …Yikes!

I wrote Wayne a poem for our 19th anniversary. I thought I would include it because it describes where we are, and how I never imagined our 19th Anniversary would be like this.

Dear Wayne,

Today we've been married
For nineteen years
We've shared lots of laughter
We've shared in the tears

We've enjoyed together
So many things
I can hardly believe
The joys your love brings!

Who could have imagined
On our wedding day
While the sun was shining
And our friends were at play

That nineteen years later
Almost right on the clock
We'd be seeing my Oncologist
Now that doesn't rock!

Through the good times and bad
All the highs and the lows
We're there for each other

Hand in hand we both go

I cannot imagine
What I'd do without you
Your warmth and your humour
Always help get me through

It seems at this moment
That our carefree days
Of laughter and sunshine
And dancing and play

Have left us so quickly
And I don't know why
I ask of the Heavens
It just makes me cry

But surely there are more
Good times in store
For our family and our love
Please tell me you're sure!

Even though these are tough days
I'm so grateful too
For the love and support
I can count on from you

To say you are fabulous
That's not enough
You're funny, sweet, and thoughtful
My hero, my rock & hot stuff!

How can I ever say
What you mean to me?
I just need to try
I hope you will see

You're my friend and lover
Of nineteen plus years
You lift me up always
You help ease my fears

You make me feel like
I can do anything
No challenge insurmountable
You make my heart sing

You're the Daddy, the Wayner
The hubby, the one that I call
To make me feel sane
And make sense of it all

You're my fixer of screen doors
My washer of floors
My gourmet chef, party boy,
Sexy pool guy, and Toy!

You are "Mr. Wonderful"
You're the world to me
Thank you for sharing
Your life with me!

I love you Wayne!
Truly, madly, deeply...
I can't wait to be 100% back so we can enjoy the rest of our lives
together!
Love you always,
Carolyn xoxoxoxoxoxoxo...

If you think you can't make a difference in someone's life, just try. It's the little things that make all the difference. It's always the little acts of kindness and thoughtfulness that meant so much to me. Some days, going through treatment, the slightest thing that brought me a smile made the world of difference. In other words, "If you think you are too small to be effective, then you've never been in bed with a mosquito." *(Bette Reese)*

Contentment

Does it seem sadistic to say that at various points during my cancer journey, I have been blessed to feel some of the most extreme feelings of contentment, that I have ever experienced before in my life? When you think about all the pain and suffering and difficulties I have faced, why how can it be that I could experience anything remotely connected to contentment? How do I feel contentment when I should feel discontent and why did I feel discontent when I should have been content?

One autumn afternoon, as I walked my dogs along Jerseyville Road, I gazed across the fields and farmlands, the soothing powder blue sky, I inhaled and was overcome with feelings of peace and contentment. Just out of the blue, it was like a wave of intangible bliss wrapped around me, and then sunk into my brain, my body, my soul, and then it soaked right through to my bones and settled comfortably there. Wow!

I have experienced this wave of contentment a few times and each time the experience is rich and powerful and completely unexpected! It surprises me and I wonder to myself, why now? Why when my world is upside down, my body is torn in so many ways from treatments, my emotions drained, my adrenaline extinguished, and then like a breath of fresh air, my lungs fill up and drink the invisible nectar of contentment and I feel so grateful to be here! I feel so grateful to be alive, for this moment, for all the blessings life has given me. I feel grateful that I can walk, I have strength, I have love, I have family and sunshine and temporarily, my entire world is blanketed in warmth, comfort and bliss!

Strangely, over the past few years of my life before breast cancer, there have been many moments of agitation, anxiousness, fear, exhaustion, frustration and discontent. When things were going really well in my life and I had my health and energy and stamina and so many other things that I felt were meaningful, I experienced amongst the happiness, many moments of discontentment. Boy, was that dumb! I had no idea! I had life so good and yet I didn't fully appreciate it! Now that I have had to face so many physical, emotional and spiritual challenges, I feel grateful for so many things I used to take for granted.

When I can reach down in the shower to shave my legs, and not feel pain, I feel grateful. When I'm driving and I can turn the steering wheel to into or get out of a tight spot, and I can do it pain free, I am happy. When I can walk freely, and when I am able to exercise without too many restrictions, I feel alive and energetic. When I can easily walk my dogs more than 2 kilometers and enjoy it, I feel very happy, especially just to be outside, enjoying the walk, the air and time to think! When I can lift the water jug or my shopping bags without the need for assistance, I feel strong and independent!

I am grateful when I can hug my husband and my children and not feel tissue expanders digging deep into my rib cage; that feels good! All of these little things, and many more, now register gratitude in my brain! I take pleasure in the little things and I don't want to take things for granted anymore! I have my cancer to thank for this enlightenment. When I experience blissful feelings of contentment during the most unimaginable trials and tribulations, my thoughts turn to say, "Thank you!"

Perhaps this is one of the lessons to be learned, that I need to find gratification in the everyday, important little things.

4 Tests & Other Freaky Stuff

"What lies behind us and what lies before us, are small matters, compared to what lies within us." (Emerson)

Mixed Feelings

I'm not sure about feeling sexy - it's all just very strange. I don't want to lose that part of my life & our relationship - Wayne & me... It's just strange. It's a mixture of feelings - but I am not fearful at the moment - well not too much! I feel mostly good and somewhat normal but every now and then I find my mind is totally preoccupied and I cannot concentrate. On Friday I felt periodically weepy, but that has been the only day so far that I have felt that way, other than the Monday when I went for all the testing & spent half the day in the hospital.

Well, truthfully it's a mixture of ~ good, pretty good, ok and kabookied out, not good and then pretty good again - all at different times. I am still surprised at how together I feel – considering what is coming up...

I'm as ready as I can be, to take on whatever comes my way. When I pray, I don't dare ask God to cure me and get rid of my cancer, but I do pray and ask him to please give me the strength and courage to deal with whatever comes my way and whatever I need to handle. I feel like I don't have the right to ask for a cure, but of course, I hope I make it. I already have plans to bake cookies with my grandchildren and take them to the park, and have fun together. Of course that is a long way off. I just hope I'm here for it, but if not, then I at least hope I am here for my children when they need me, for at least until they are in their 20's.

First Surgeon's Opinion

Wayne & I were in pretty good spirits, all things considered. The last time I spent any time in St. Joseph's Hospital was for a D&C after miscarriage of our first baby, back in 1994. Although that definitely crossed my mind, this was a completely different adventure! We went up to Dr. Loverick's waiting room and were soon escorted into his tiny examining room. Really being somewhat strangers to hospitals, we passed the time by being silly. Wayne always has a great sense of humour, and it has helped us in many situations! For now, this awkward situation was no different. I was wearing one of those terribly sexy, faded pale blue, slightly visible plaid print, terribly terrible hospital gowns with the fabric ties at the neck and the middle, but this time I had it open to the front and not the back. When Dr. Lovericks talked we listened intently, and what we were hearing was very intense! We tried to take it all in but it was overwhelming. It was surreal that this could be happening. When he turned his back toward me for a moment or when he left the room, that is when we somehow found it in us to misbehave. We felt like a couple of silly kids, coping with the news of cancer, the only way we knew how. When Dr. Lovericks turned his back to draw a picture or how my boob would be cut, I quickly flashed Wayne my boobs! When Dr. Lovericks looked away, I looked at Wayne and made suggestive faces and gestures with my tongue. He did the same to me, when the doctor wasn't looking. When the doctor left the room, Wayne got on the scale, he played with his instruments, and looked in the drawers of the examining table. It was ridiculous, but we were nervous and we weren't ready to cope with the seriousness of our situation. Misbehaving in the doctor's office was indicative of the early days and our naive hopes that things could be normal. Somehow we managed to still be playful and laughter soothed both of our nerves, for a little while.

We met with Dr. Peter Lovericks, my first impression was that he was definitely a man I could trust. He was very caring, sensitive and thorough. He explained things well and I was able to keep my thoughts from panic, as he went through what kind of surgery he would do. Dr. Lovericks suggested that he would recommend that I have chemotherapy first to see if they can shrink the tumors, known as adjuvant chemotherapy, but Wayne & I talked about it. I was of the mindset that I just wanted to have the cancer taken out of my body. Every day I lived as its host, I felt a bit creeped out. I wondered what it was feeding on, and where it was having a party, without my knowledge! I saw it as an insidious, rude house guest, sneaking around and going wild, all the while, making a huge mess inside my body, wreaking havoc and trying to ruin my life and yet, despite all the mess it created, I end up having to go the great lengths to clean it all up! I wanted it out – the sooner the better!

I would feel better if the cancer was gone first and then I could have chemo to poison the stragglers, if there are any! Plus I will get to keep my hair a little longer. I am really scared about chemo. Because of this decision, we went for another opinion with Dr. Saunders. I was thinking that whoever could get me to surgery first, would be the surgeon I would go with. That turned out to be Dr. Saunders.

The Days before Treatments Begin: May 3, 2009

Wow, where has the time gone? Tomorrow morning I will have an MRI at the Henderson Hospital at 8:15. Then I will have an appointment with Dr. Ken Saunders (no relation to "Kernel/Colonel Saunders" of KFC, as far as I know! - Thankfully) at 1:00pm. I am feeling anxious to get started but on the same thought, I will likely look back on these days before treatments, as the last "golden days" of feeling kind of "normal"! I don't want to wish any time away, that is for sure. However, I am scared about what the cancer is doing while I am busy waiting for things to happen and get appointments going. Already I can feel the largest mass is larger. It is definitely wider and the shape of my breast has changed, to more of a teardrop shape. Also my nipple is almost completely sucked in now, which looks so strange. I wonder how much further it will go. I do feel some tenderness and a little discomfort when the seatbelt pushes against my breast, and at some other times too.

I think I might be okay with the MRI tomorrow. I am claustrophobic, but maybe, just maybe, I will be able to look past this hurdle to the bigger picture. I actually WANT to know what is going on inside me, unlike the last time I had an MRI about 4 or 5 years ago, and I was very afraid of what might be found in my head... Time will tell, I guess.

 I finished up work on Friday, May 1. It is not a good feeling not to have my job, but I know I have to let it go, to focus on my health. As well, I am determined to get my Coop Part 3 (Specialist) course finished by Friday! I want it out of the way and done!

I want to include all about my last week at work and the people who have been so wonderful to me but for how I have to crash!

MRI – Stick Your Tits in This Hole & Don't Move!

I've only ever had one previous MRI and being claustrophobic, I was not looking forward to repeating the experience! The first time it was to check things out regarding my headaches and I was very nervous. I was shaking so badly by the time I waited the 2+ hours in the waiting room, that there was no way I could possibly be still. I was a wreck. They injected me with the drugs and somehow I got through it. I don't recall that I actually stopped physically shaking, but I must have. I don't know what made me so nervous, but I can tell you that at the time, I felt absolutely terrified. It seems stupid when I look back now, but in the moment, it was brutal!

Well, there's one thing about being faced with breast cancer that changes your outlook on things. I think this is healthy. Suddenly, things that used to scare the wits out of me now, by comparison, seem much smaller and manageable.

Sunday night, before my MRI, I was expecting to feel those too familiar butterflies. They didn't come. I wondered when (if) I would be nervous about this MRI because I wasn't feeling it at all. My thoughts were occupied by the bigger picture – having breast cancer. The MRI didn't feel like such a big deal. It was just one more thing to go through on the journey...

When I was called in, I felt a few butterflies. I was asked to sit in a big comfy chair by a super sweet nurse who made me feel so at ease – like it was all manageable! I took some comfort from her reassuring attitude and it actually occurred to me that I would be able to manage the MRI this time! She put an IV in my arm and explained what would happen. I gazed around the room at a few other patients, waiting their turn for a CT scan or an MRI or whatever. I was, by far, the youngest one there!! My angel nurse explained that they would be injecting a dye into me at a certain point and that I would feel a cold sensation and I might taste something funny. Everything happened exactly as she explained!

The funny thing was my instructions. On the MRI table, I had to lay on my stomach and there was a small hole covered in sheets, just large enough for my boobs to fall into. They told me to put my breasts in there and do not move! The funny thing was, I was concentrating very hard on not moving but I was very conscious of my chest rising and falling because of my breathing. I lay there, my hair pulled back from tickling my face, ear plugs inserted, headphones on playing music and my tits hanging vulnerably like unsuspecting udders of a cow, about to be milked. I didn't know if I would feel anything going across my breasts. I tried to take shallow breaths, but I needed to breathe. I shut my eyes tightly and tried to make my mind go back to the beach in Jamaica! That kind of helped. The machine clunked, banged, groaned, hammered and clanged away. I tried to be patient and thought about my yoga training. I got through it! I was dizzy when I got up but otherwise, unscathed! I felt a new sense of confidence rising within me and I felt proud of myself for "mastering" the machine! I was grateful to see Wayne at the end of it and I enjoyed the slight feeling of empowerment for a little while! It lasted until we met with my surgeon, Dr. Ken Sanders later that afternoon!

Modified Radical Mastectomy

On May 7, 2009, I made my obligatory appearance at the Henderson Hospital. I still found it strange for me to be the one who was the patient. I felt fine physically, but emotionally, I was not fine at all. I wanted drugs to chill me out. I followed the directions ~ go here, go there, wait there… I obediently, passively and yet nervously went through the motions until I was situated in a chair behind a curtain, waiting for the nurse to come and put an I.V. in me. The "no-nonsense nurse" made her early morning grim appearance, said nothing, and proceeded to slap me hard on the back of my left hand. It hurt too. I couldn't help but feel she was taking out her frustrations on me. I told her that she wouldn't likely be able to find a vein there.

Rather oblivious to me, and hell-bent on her mission, she continued to smack my hand hard, and search for a vein. I pull my hand away and she begins to consider the idea that I might actually be right. She has a look at my left arm and decides she needs to call for the "I.V. nurse." I am a little relieved to be free from her abusive, disregarding methods but I do want to get this nastiness over with. Shortly another nurse appears around the curtain and she spies the only visible vein in the crook of my left arm. One good attempt and she has the I.V. in place. Of course, it hurts, but I know that soon I won't feel anything and at least this part of the ordeal is past.

I'm feeling like more of a "sick" person with a hospital gown on and an I.V. stuck in my arm now. Wayne and I share a little conversation and I am truly scared! I don't want to have cancer. I feel well. I don't feel sick. I don't want to have to lose my breast, but I know it is all going to happen and I have to deal with it and accept it. Still, it's very scary. Tears only come once and I blink them back. Sometimes I turn to humour for comfort. I reach into my bag for the stickers I had prepared, just for this occasion.

Me trying to still be me!

Before I went into surgery I decided to put labels on my tits. Besides the fact that I wanted to inject a little humour into such a serious experience in my life, I also wanted to try & connect with the staff in the "OR" who would be taking care of me. I didn't want them to see me as just a deadweight body. I wanted them to see me as a person. As well, I didn't want to take any chances of getting the wrong breast removed. I wrote little notes on sticky labels and stuck them on my tits. The notes read:

Left Breast:
Dear Dr. Saunders,
Please leave this breast. (LEFT) The other one is the one with the cancer. Thank you!
Carolyn xo

Right Breast:
Dear Dr. Saunders and your team of Angels,
Thank you for taking care of me! This breast is the one with the
cancer. (RIGHT) You can take it. Thank you for your TLC!
Love Carolyn xoxo

The Operating Room

I walked down the hall and into the Operating Room. Everything seemed cast by a greenish light and it was all very blurry, in particular, because I did not have my glasses on. I wasn't sure if I was grateful for that, but I think I was! I climbed onto the bed in the very chilly operating room and laid down. It was freezing. I wanted to be anywhere but here! I just wanted it to be over. I felt quite sentimental and a little distraught about my last moments with both breasts. They had always been a great source of pleasure and I knew when I woke up, that one would be gone forever. It was not a happy thought. I re-focused on the immediate, talking light-heartedly with the nurses and wondering if that fuzzy looking tall, male was my surgeon. Yes, he was Dr. Saunders. It was happening... There was no turning back.

Before I was under the anesthetic, the nurses saw the label on my left breast and chuckled, so I was happy. Since the room was freezing my body was shaking and I was shivering, but a moment later, I was out.

The "Recovery" Room

My next waking moment I found that I was in the scary recovery room. I had no idea what had transpired but my body felt tight and sore and I was feeling a severe fogginess in my brain. My throat was incredibly dry and I desperately wanted some water and someone to talk to. I checked – yes, sure enough, it was over. My right breast was gone and there were tubes coming out my right side somewhere in the vicinity of where my right breast used to live happily.

A lot of things happened to me in recovery, but it all remains a "bits & pieces" kind of memory. The sequence in which everything happened could be distorted. Overall, I felt extremely vulnerable, lonely and very afraid. My husband was there with me but I understood that it was some kind of privilege having him in there, as people are not usually allowed any visitors in the recovery room. There were so many beds in there but I had a vague awareness that many people were being moved out by the time the evening progressed. I was not one of them. What I didn't realize at that point, was that there was no room available for me! One of the first things I wanted was to see my husband and I was so afraid, I wanted him to stay with me. Thankfully, he was there when I came into some form of consciousness. It is such a surreal feeling – am I really here? Did the surgery happen? Is it over? What is wrong with me? Can I drink? I am so thirsty. Where are my children? When can they come in to see me? Etc.

My children were not allowed to see me in the "recovery" room and I felt quite devastated and indignant about this decision. Sadly, in my state of post op, all I could do was weakly cry. Wayne brought me in a photo of the kids in a plastic Ziplock bag, so I could tape it to my bed, so that was how I saw my children. When it came time for Wayne to leave, I felt truly devastated and alone! I pleaded with him not to go. I was quite honestly terrified! They basically kicked him out! One caring nurse, asked why I was crying. Before I could respond, overwhelmed with emotion and having extreme difficulty speaking because of feeling a very dry, sore throat from the surgery, the nasty nurse named Ursula responded for me, "Oh, she's just upset because her husband had to leave!" Her tone was so dismissive I felt like a child who had just peed her pants. It was so insulting and degrading that I was so infuriated that I just felt a whole lot worse. The emotions were complex and how could Nurse Nasty know why I was crying – sure that was one of the sixteen reasons, but I was pissed off! I wanted to forcefully, demand, "How dare you?!", but I was in no state to say any such thing. Not only did I feel like crap, but I was so vulnerable and at their mercy! Who the hell did she think she was?! It made me feel so much worse, and vulnerable for being there! It was horrible!

One of the caring nurses came over to check on me, Heady, and was alarmed to find out that one of my drains in my side was leaking and I was laying in a pool of blood! Apparently Nurse Nasty was supposed to be looking out for me, but somehow she missed that! I don't think she came close enough to me to check anything. Hmmm... The last time Nurse Nasty looked at me, she told me, there is no point in giving me morphine for the pain, as I couldn't take it home with me. She said , "You're going home tonight, and you can't take the morphine with you!" (Tylenol does nothing for me. It never has!) Of course, before I could say anything she is shoving 2 Tylenol 3, at me in the tiniest paper cup I have ever seen. No water of course. While she is shoving the pills at me at the full extent of her arm, she is looking in another direction, avoiding eye contact. She doesn't even stop by my bed but continues on to another patient or something I couldn't see. In a few seconds she is back in my vicinity, but not exactly next to my bed, only to ask authoritatively, "What, you haven't taken the pills yet?!" with the tone of what kind of moron are you! I manage a squeak, "I need some water to take them". Disgruntled, she sashays off to reluctantly get me some water. I feel like sarcastically saying, "Sorry to inconvenience you!" but I cannot muster it up at all. I am too sick & vulnerable to do much of anything. I think to myself, "Man, I just lost my breast, I was perfectly fine yesterday before I came here. I have to face chemotherapy and cancer soon and I'm going to even lose my hair, and you think it's okay to treat me like shit. Unbelievable!" Again I feel even worse – if that is even possible!

The caring nurse Heady, checks in on me and asks me about my pain, on a scale of 1 to 10. I tell her it's about 8. She says "There is no need for you to have pain, my dear." She returns to top up my IV with morphine and I feel the relief almost immediately as the elixir rushes through my veins. Caring Nurse checks my bandages and my drains and discovers to her horror that I am lying in a pool of blood. She sees that my drains have been leaking and she is very concerned. Caring Nurse, who I now totally regard as my Guardian Angel, also notices that something is growing on my chest – what I later found out to be a hematoma. At this point she seemed to make it her mission to take care of me. Thank God, I pray. She was just the angel I so desperately needed!

Oh what a Curtain can do – Nothing!

Despite all the indignities of the so-called "Recovery Room", another thing that scared me was what I could hear! My bed just happened to be right next to the Nurses desk, and there was only a curtain between us. Perhaps they forgot that although I could not see them, I could certainly hear through that curtain! *"I can't wait to get out of here!" "I can't retire soon enough." "I hope there will be something left of me by the time I get out of here." "The docs don't care." "My husband wants me to retire now. He's worried about what will happen to me if I stay in this job much longer." "This job is killing me!" "Oh, what do they want now?" "This is ridiculous." "I can't wait to get out of here! I'm NOT staying late. I don't care where they (patients) go, but I'm not staying here!" They (the Docs) have no idea." "He's a pain in the ass." (a patient)* The overall feelings of despair, exhaustion, diminished, hopelessness, obvious burn out and negativity, coming from staff behind the curtain, only filled me with more dread and trepidation! If I had been able I would have stuck my fingers in my ears and blocked out their appalling conversations with a hefty "La-la-la-la-la-la…!" but I was in no shape to save myself from the anguishing assaults of their uncaring, selfish, petrifying words. I was truly a victim, feeling like I was on the edge of life and death, dependent on their "care" for my every function! I layed there in the "Recovery Room" wondering if it wouldn't just be better to "slip away" beyond this room and beyond this existence into the next life, and not cause these poor nurses any more suffering. I felt utterly vulnerable and completely at their mercy.

Wow, some things patients just were NOT meant to hear!

I won't reveal all of the gory details, but I can say that these were some of the most unhappy, disgruntled, negative, bad attitude, overworked, under-appreciated, supposedly professional people, I had ever encountered. They talked amongst themselves about how their bodies were not able to cope with the stress and strain of the demands of their job, how they couldn't "get out" fast enough. How much they hated the job, how patients sucked the life out of them, how no one cared about them, how much shit they had to deal with, how no one outside Recovery understands their plight, how thankless and unappreciated they felt, etc, etc., etc.

There are many things that a patient should not hear and I wished that I didn't have to hear what I heard. Don't get me wrong, I have EVERY respect for Nurses! If I had the guts, I would have loved to become a Nurse. They have long hours, they work hard and they have such a critical, consequential and righteous role, in the lives of those who need them! I love to help people and it seems to me that this is the paramount mission of any nurse. They have my utmost respect and admiration, however, I wish I was not privy to what I heard in the Recovery room that night. I've made a point not to base any future thoughts of Nurses on what I was so devastated to hear.

I heard my Angel Nurse firmly telling another nurse, who was arguing with her, that she was going to stay beyond her shift to take care of me. I got the impression that no one was supposed to be in the recovery room all night, as we were all supposed to have beds elsewhere in the hospital, but that was not going to happen. There was one other man, and me, who didn't have anywhere to go, and I was still in rough shape. My Angel Nurse told the other nurse that she was going to stay and that was that. I heard one nurse telling my Angel Nurse that she was to leave at 11:30 when her shift ended. Angel Nurse said she was staying until at least 3:30 and perhaps longer if necessary, and thank God, she did just that.

I remember the urge when I felt I needed to go pee. I wanted to get up and get out of bed to go but they said I couldn't as long as I was in the "recovery room". They said I had to stay in bed. They offered me a bed pan. Hmmm... Have you ever tried to go pee when you are laying down? My brain would not permit my bladder to release. I tried and tried, but nothing, although the necessity to "go" was strong. They closed the curtain and still, nothing was happening as long as I was horizontal. Then they said I could sit up a bit in bed. They cranked the top half of the bed to a semi vertical position and I suddenly felt gravely ill. I felt a heavy cloud of darkness come sweeping over me, from the top of my head downward and I barely had time to speak or even think a full thought. I thought that perhaps this was the end and I felt incredibly dire, as my body plunged and then crashed into a deep puddle of blackness. Everything around me was consumed by the blackness. The next thing I knew, there were lots of people around me, fussing and talking and trying to get my attention. I could hear them, but although they were beside me, they seemed so far away. I could see them all around the bed. I could feel their urgency, but I had no idea what they were doing to my body. I certainly could not speak to them with my voice. My voice was nowhere to be found. I really had no idea what happened, but I vaguely knew I was no longer sinking in the black puddle that had consumed me. I heard them saying "she crashed, low blood pressure, passed out" and before I knew anything else, I was back into a completely horizontal position, and feeling a wee bit grateful for that.

I think they relieved me with a catheter at that point. It's a blur.

Later that evening, I remember my Angel Nurse, and another sweet Nurse named Heather or Nicole, helping me sit up and washing my back, my neck and my face with nice warm water. They carefully and respectfully dried me off and I felt so much better.

In the morning, the shift changed and I was very relieved not to see Nurse Nasty in the crew! Although I could still sense tension amongst the day sift of nurses and I could feel stabs of bitchiness coming through in their conversations. Nothing I heard that morning seemed to be directed at the patients, just at each other. There were some derogatory comments and snide remarks about who was there before them and what was done & not done from the night before. A young, newish to the "Recovery Room" Nurse, named Crystal, seemed to be the target for one of the older nasty nurses that morning. I wanted so much to save Crystal from her wrath and in a different situation, I would have come to her defense.

I still wanted to get up and go to the washroom and I finally persuaded them to let me get out of bed to go, as the bedpan was not working for me. I managed to get Crystal to take me out of the room and down the hall in a wheel chair, so I could go pee. We took our time and chatted and it was such a relief to be out of that room! I gave Crystal what encouragement I could. I could tell she was a good nurse and a good person and I didn't want her to feel beaten down, discouraged or diminished by the Nasty nurse so I told her everything good I had observed about her, that morning. Getting out of there just to go to the bathroom was the best break I had had! I think it helped both of us.

Dr. Saunders came in to check on me. I know he had a golf game planned, for that afternoon, but he was keeping an eye on the hematoma that was developing on my chest. My first thought was, "Oh, I'm growing another boob already!" Not exactly... Dr, Saunders was concerned that he would need to operate again to seal it off. Sure enough, in no time, the hematoma had grown larger than a golf ball on the right side of my chest where my breast used to live. I happily waved good bye to the Recovery Room staff, pleased to be getting out of there. I jokingly told them, on my way out, "I'm gonna miss this place!" and "It's been a slice." As I was rolled out to a room on a ward. Finally, they had a room for me, but it was very short lived. Before lunch time that day, I ended up back in surgery, anesthetic all over again, my mastectomy scar re-opened and the hematoma taken care of. Before I knew it I was back in the dreaded "Recovery Room" again! The same staff was there whom I had joked with earlier that day. I told them I was only joking when I said, "I'm gonna miss this place!" a few hours earlier! They chuckled and I found the "Recovery Room" wasn't quite as dreadful the second time in less than 24 hours, and I was soon sent to a room for 4 on a ward.

Bone Scan – Coffin Simulator
June 17, 2009

Today is my brother Greg's 41st birthday. He & his family are going whale watching in St. Andrews. I'm so happy for them! I didn't tell him that my bone scan was today. I didn't want to think about that on his birthday. You may remember I am not good with claustrophobia. I don't like to be in confined spaces when I feel out of control. Of course I feel very comfy in airplanes and totally fine in elevators but inside of machines when my movement is restricted in some way – that is not my idea of a good time. I don't know why it is so silly that it causes me stress. I used to have this recurring dream when I was a child. I would wake up in a panic every time. I would be in a crawl space, like a chimney or a box and I could not turn around. It was cramped and stuffy and every time I would freak out!!! I felt like I couldn't breathe. I hated it! I still hate the idea, but of course, I wouldn't go into a crawl space for pretty much anything.

Wayne took me into the hospital. So I got the injection of radioactive isotopes and felt just fine. I went out to lunch with Colleen to Cora's and that was a wonderful diversion. I love Cora's and I love talking to Colleen. She is so understanding and non judgmental. She asks a lot of questions too – like she really gets it. That was the good part of my day.

So I get back to the hospital and wait for my turn in the bone scan machine. A tiny Asian female technician comes out to get me and she looks like about 12 years old. Very cute. Very young. I think she is a student. A male technician sits further back to watch the computer while the scanner does its thing on me. I love my jewelry and I don't like having to take off my wedding rings especially. It's too much of my identity. I don't want to be uncooperative though so I do as I am instructed. I will do whatever it takes. I remove the last of my jewelry and my glasses and climb on the table. I ask the tiny Asian girl a lot of questions – how long will it take? How close will it come to my face? Will it scan my head? Do I have to stay still? Will I feel anything? Can they see anything on the computer screen? Can I talk? Thoughtfully she senses my anxious feelings and offers to sit beside me on a chair as the scanner goes over my head to talk me through it. Surprisingly, it helps. Just the conversation helps. I feel slightly less weird. She straps my feet together so they cannot move. She straps me into/onto the table and I resign myself to the loss of control. I try to calm my thoughts. I feel the machine moving all around – up & down. I put the brakes on my thoughts that it might malfunction and crush me right then &

there. Phew! I admit I am claustrophobic and a little worried. The tiny little one tries to console me. I ask if she has ever been in the bone scan machine. She says she has in school. It doesn't bother her. It bothers me.

We get started. I close my eyes afraid of what the visual will do to my stress level. The machine comes down to my forehead and is a fraction off my nose. Briefly I contemplate what I will do if it continues any closer. I will freak! I barely dare open my eyes because I can feel my breath right back on my nose as I exhale because the scan is so close. I think to myself – this is a coffin simulator. I don't want to think about it but that is all I can think of. As the scanner gradually works its way down my body and my face is out of its range, I breathe a temporary little sign of relief. Once it is past my face, I can talk and ask questions again. I ask a few more. The male technician is not budging. I wonder what he is looking at. Why does he have to look at my body this way? Do I look like a sick person to him? Can he see cancer having a party in my body and he won't tell me? I kind of resent the fact that he will not communicate with me at all. At the end he just smiles – and not a good smile just an icky smile. It has taken over an hour because I drank all the fluid they asked me to and I need to go out part way through and empty my bladder again. Being nervous didn't help.

Before I leave I ask again if they saw anything. The tiny Asian girl says they say my bones & my bladder and the radioactive dye. Hmmm… nothing is going to give here. I ask when Dr. Arnold will have the results of the test. I resign myself to the fact that I am not going to crack these two.

I leave to find out that Victoria has had a very rough orthodontist appointment and she is crying and upset. I am later than I thought I would be but I do manage, despite the 403 dinner time traffic, to meet Wayne & Toria on Hamilton Drive so I can take her to her last Jazz class of the year. She is happier about that. I am feeling a bit tired and hungry but Victoria is more important to me. We get a bite to eat at Tim Horton's afterward so she is feeling happier, by the time her class is finished. I am very, very tired.

Ultrasound

There are a lot of tests to go through once you have a cancer diagnosis. Besides, the initial mammogram, breast ultrasound, biopsy, numerous blood tests, bone scan, radioactive dye injections, breast MRI and chest x-ray, there is also the abdominal ultrasound. Like a lot of women, we are familiar with ultrasounds because it was something we were usually very happy to have when we we're pregnant, so we could sneak a peek at our wee one and perhaps even get a trick, a flip or a wave from them! The hardest part was holding in those 5-6 gallons of water we were required to drink, 15 minutes before! I learned that an abdominal ultrasound to search for cancer metastasis is not quite as exciting and there is no "show & tell" component. To someone like me, this can be very disconcerting. Right from the start I wanted to see everything. I wanted to know everything and I wanted to know it now! I wanted to face it up front, head on, with balls and a determined attitude. Needless to say, for this ultrasound, I was left to employ my powers of feminine intuition to read the faces and gestures and every little detail of the trained professionals who practice their poker faces every day, for a living. At least I didn't have to drink gallons of water and try to hold my pee in for this one.

Right from the start, as the younger technician began with the slimy goo on my abdomen below my breast, and mastectomy scar, it was all serious, hard pushing. No smiles, no small talk, no jokes, no sideway glances. She scanned me inch by inch and I was not able to see the screen, despite how much I craned my neck. The experienced supervisor kept a watchful eye, and then suddenly I saw it: the questioning look on the young technician's face. Confirmation: the supervisor took over the chair and the controls and I detected a slight variation in her well-established poker face. It was so subtle. Next thing I knew she was pushing me very hard deep into the right side of my abdomen. She was saying "Sorry, I'm so sorry, I just have to get this," as she pushed and pushed the doppler hard into me. My mind raced about, trying to pinpoint what organ they were looking at. I scolded myself for not remembering more of Biology and anatomy, but I couldn't help but tune in to my feminine intuition. I think the technician found something "questionable" on my liver. I thought, it must be my liver she was trying to capture a closer picture of. Breast cancer has its favourite party spots in the body. It prefers to branch out to the lungs, the brain and the liver, but it will go just about anywhere it can.

The whole thing was unsettling, but truthfully at that time, I had no idea just how serious my battle for life would have been, if the party had spread to my liver. Even though I asked what they saw and what they were looking at, etc. I had to wait for the results to hear that it was my gall bladder they were photographing and it had a few polyps on it. No big deal. When Wayne found this out, he almost cried. Tears came to his eyes and he was so relieved. I really didn't grasp the potential danger that would have meant, but he did!

All of these tests were all part of determining the staging of the cancer. After all, it turned out that my cancer was staged at 3A.

Not what I expected, but how would I know!

I learned a lot after surgery. There were many frustrations that I did not expect! I didn't know that it would be so hard to use and move my right arm. Reaching up, down or reaching at all, was challenging! It hurt like heck. I thought I wasn't supposed to do any exercises until I at least had the drains removed, but after a follow up visit with Dr. Saunders, I learned I was wrong. There is so much going on when you have surgery and are faced with a cancer diagnosis, that they can't possibly prepare you for everything, I guess. What I wished someone had mentioned and emphasized was the need for physiotherapy, as soon as possible. When I saw Dr. Saunders, a week or 2 after surgery, one of the things he asked me to do was to raise my arm. I proudly raised my arm out to the front, level with my shoulder, and there it came to an abrupt stop. He bluntly said, "No. Raise your arm." That was it. It was as raised as I could get it to go. He abruptly said, you better start exercising that arm or you are going to lose your mobility and it will be cemented there. Wow, not such a delicate way of putting things, so I knew I had to start working on it right away.

Simple little things were very difficult. Trying to squish the soap dispenser to get the soap out was painful, trying to open a child-proof medicine jar, opening doors, turning on taps, trying to grasp the seatbelt and pull it across my body, scratching an itch, reaching for anything, was all painful in varying degrees. I felt like a cord was shortened in my armpit and I could no longer reach. I could no longer reach above my head or behind my back. Small motor skills were very challenging, like brushing my hair, pouring a cup of tea, and simply taking the cap off the toothpaste were now things that were challenging to me, because of the surgery. I started physiotherapy and the work and exercises were a tremendous help, but as the summer went on and I endured chemo, I found I no longer had the energy or desire to commit to physiotherapy, but still it helped me regain most of my mobility! This gave me a small glimpse of how tough it must be for the elderly.

Sleeping comfortably was difficult. I could only sleep on my back, not my side and obviously not my stomach. VON Nurses came and went daily, out of my house, checking on me, changing and cleaning my wounds, charting my progress, answering my questions, and some taking time to chat and connect with me as a person. Overall, there were a lovely, caring collection of ladies, and I really appreciated their care.

Any Port will do! (...in a storm!)

The hospital is so quiet in the main outpatient areas before 8am. I like it that way. As I always feel that I absorb the emotions of others, I find it less draining to be there when there is relatively no one around. I find my way through to the Special Procedures area of radiology & ultrasound. I am the only soul in the stuffy waiting room which has a ceiling fan whirling stale air and a completely sealed window that looks out into a triangular space filled with construction debris and two solid walls. Couldn't be less interesting I think to myself. I am nervous about the procedure and I wonder how long I will have to wait, and what will happen. I just want it to be over! Wayne has gone to take Victoria to Katie's for the morning so we don't have to worry about any sibling issues between them. One less stress. I reluctantly sit alone and still, all is quiet.

Amanda, a young nurse or technician came in to get me. My instincts are still telling me to run! Run fast, run far – escape – get out of here. I understand the logic of the port and I do think it is a good idea overall, but one more thing to get poked in me, another cut, more anesthetic, more stitches, more ickiness, more ouch. It creeps me out – having a foreign device implanted in my chest. I try not to think about it. I worry about the IV for the surgery. I worry that I will be awake – yikes, how creepy is that!!!! Even now, thinking back to the experience, my mind really prefers to block what it knows and deny it ever happened.

A nurse named Pat, very pleasant, gets me ready for the procedure. She puts in the IV – ugh another.... And she and Amanda work away at what they need to do, while waiting & wondering where the doctor is and when he will show up to get started. Even with the IV, I still have the urge to run away!

Wayne sits with me while. I wait, passively, helplessly, I wait for my fate. I try to keep a brave face but I feel weak. He is strong for me and uses his warmth and humour to try and ease my stress. I admire that he tries but I am not in the mood to be cajoled. I am feeling too real too raw and too sentimental and yet I must not break down. We talk and reminisce about how we were at the Henderson Hospital 14 years ago on this day, for Wesley's birth. Who could have known that 14 years later we would be back but for me going through breast cancer?! I tell Wayne, "I just want this all to be over" Wayne thinks I am referring to the port installation procedure. Although that is included in what I want to be OVER, I am actually referring to the big picture – it ALL! All the chemo, all the IV, all the surgery and recovery anal the hair loss and regrowth, ALL the ickiness! All of it! How am I going to cope when I feel like I am done and this is only the beginning? I just don't know how...

Dr. Torbiak makes his entrance, late but seemingly unfrazzeled! He is tall, built, handsome, trendy and very sexy. The term "maverick" comes to my mind. I will be in his care. Already I am feeling a wee bit better about the prospect of getting this port stuck inside me. We chat, he reassures me and makes me feel he has everything under complete control. It's how I want to feel.

I am awake as the procedure requires. They have given me the drug I nick –name "IDGAS" and I am one happy camper. Everything is just fine! My thoughts wander, as they always do, and I think, "Sure they can saw off my leg, as long as they put it back. I'm okay with that!" Crazy! Dr. Flipping Gorgeous asks me what kind of music I like. We agree that we both love "The Police" and he starts the procedure to the sultry music of, "Roxanne"...you don't need to turn on that red light..." and I am happy!

Everything goes well, but the sensations are exceptionally odd! Now I think I know how a fish must feel when hooked on a fishing line. (minus the obvious panic, in the fish's case) They pull a wire or a string or whatever, through my neck and thread it down into my chest and my heart arteries as it needs to go. All I needed to do was lay there and breathe as they instructed me to. Easy assignment. In what seemed like about 20 minutes, I was lying down in a recovery room with "tag-o-derm" over where my port was placed and where I was stitched up.

The nurse gave me some papers to assure me that home health care would be checking in on me and would be changing my dressing daily and I would be released to live happily ever after. (even without Dr. Gorgeous)

Port Removal Surgery
November 23, 2009

Well today was the much anticipated day to finally get my power port removed! I am definitely not the text book case when it comes to my port! It's not supposed to hurt. It hurt! I was supposed to get home care to change my dressings and take care of the surgery. They never came. I wasn't supposed to get cellulitis. I did. It hurt like hell. Every step was excruciatingly painful. At night when I was trying to sleep, sometimes I rolled over and the discomfort of the port sticking in my chest woke me up. I learned to roll a corner of the pillow around to protect the tender area where my port was living. When I walked, I could feel a kind of scraping inside my chest wall as it felt like it scraped with the motion of each footstep! July to November – well, that was a lot of footsteps! My bra straps irritated my chest where the port was living. The seatbelt irritated that spot! I used a little pillow underneath the seatbelt to ease the discomfort. Every day I sprayed the area with "Bactine" to take advantage of the local anesthetic quality to ease the pain & discomfort. When I got out of the shower each morning I would spray the area with "Bactine." I would repeat this for a tiny bit of relief at different times daily but always again before bed to try & ease the pain of it. Every time I got chemo, the insertion and removal of the push pin type "needle" was a killer. Most nurses looked at me in disbelief when I let out a yelp or a cry. They usually questioned me, in an obviously surprised tone, "Did that hurt?!" Although I loved the nurses and staff there and can never speak highly enough of them, this is the one thing that I never understood. I thought each time, "Do you think I yelp, wince or cry out loud, just for fun!" Hmmm... Of course it HURTS! I wouldn't just make this up!

Today I was honestly scared and nervous, not knowing what to expect and feeling a little "gun-shy" from my initial experience getting the port installed. It gave me the creeps, being awake for the surgery and feeling the pulling and tugging of "things" (veins, ligaments, and who knows what else!) in and out of my neck. I felt the cool sensation when part of my chest wall was cut open. I felt the separation of my skin but not the pain of this. It was weird and creepy. I heard the music in the Operating Room as we began, "Roxanne" by the Police. Surprisingly I still love that song! Throughout, they instructed me to breathe, and inhale or exhale, which I dutifully obeyed, while they dug around in my neck & chest. Weird!

Today there was no IV to insert. Emily the nurse told me I just needed to have local anesthetic. I was kind of hoping for that drug they gave me last time. I don't know what it was called, but I affectionately refer to it as the "I don't give a shit" (IDGAS) drug. Honesty, it was not euphoric at all, but it certainly chilled me out. They could have done anything to me, and at the time, I would have been okay with it. It totally chased away my initial extreme feelings of wanting to run away! I wish I could have had that "I don't give a shit" drug with this surgery! Emily assured me with her sweet, warm and confident smile that all would be okay and this was a procedure that not even any recovery was required. I wanted to be reassured. I wanted it to be over. I wanted the "I don't give a shit" drug. She insinuated that I definitely wouldn't need it. Emily said that since my port had only been in place since July, it shouldn't be difficult to remove. I wanted to believe her.

Dr. Chow came in to prep me. She used gauze on tongs to wipe me within a radius of what seemed like 2 feet, with pink coloured antiseptic that I swear came directly from the refrigerator and it smelled worse than 140 proof Newfie Screech. The alcohol smell was so intense it made my eyes water! Then she began to inject me with the local anesthetic. Yewouch! Man, those needles hurt! I am convinced that I have a very sensitive skin type and my freckled, fair, Irish skin means I bleed easily and I feel everything big time! Maybe I have extra nerve endings. I don't know! Well, I truly felt the full brunt of the first 3 needles and then as the anesthetic started to take affect, it became more bearable. It was hard not to be tense. Dr. Chow assured me to tell her if I felt any discomfort from what she was doing. My stomach, my back, neck and even my butt felt tight and wound. Dr. Chow made several injections of the anesthetic all around where she would be working and I felt the needle going in at least a dozen spots but at least the pain had subsided. I felt the incision and the coolness that goes with the opening and separation of my flesh. Then I felt the digging around which I presumed was to locate the nylon stitches that had secured the port in position. I felt a snip and a release, then more pulling and digging. Dr. Chow told me it was "like delivering a tiny little baby" and she didn't want to "make the incision any larger that she needed". Finally it seemed, the port was pulled out and I felt the release. She pressed on my vein to help it stop bleeding and then asked if I wanted to see it. I thought she meant my incision and the hole in my chest so I said "Yes!" Then as she reached over, behind her, I realized she was not reaching for a mirror, but for the actual port. I looked at my "tiny, little baby" that had just been delivered from my chest. It looked as I had expected. It was anti-climactic. I feigned some interest, more for the doctor's sake. I didn't want to seem unappreciative of her efforts. I really would have preferred to see the hole in my chest where that port had been camping, but I didn't say anything. I just wanted it to be over.

I figured the stitches would be easy and pain-free, since I was well frozen. Well, that is not exactly how it worked out. The first 2 or 3 stitches were okay but then suddenly the pain hit me. I felt everything – the needle, the sutcher material, the PAIN! I let out a loud wail. Dr. Chow was surprised, and asked me if I felt that. Again, I thought this was a funny thing to ask me, because I don't know that people randomly wail or react this way, if they are not in pain. Did she think I was making it up? Well, at least she listened and was apologetic and sympathetic. She injected me with more anesthetic with at least 4 more needles. She explained that possibly it was the scar tissue that had formed from the initial surgery that prevented the drugs from spreading out like they should have. She said perhaps it was because the skin had thickened because of the cellulitis that had developed post surgery. Perhaps it was my skin type – that I was more sensitive. Perhaps this was a sensitive area for me. She told me the "squelching sound was air she was pushing out of my chest from where the port had been" living. She said my skin was very "oozey" and then she explained that it was because there was a good blood supply which meant that it would heal well. Every time she told me in the surprised tone that I was so "oozey" she didn't sound like that was such a positive or normal thing.

I wanted to be done. I wanted the "I don't give a shit" drug. I suggested to Dr. Chow that I really liked the drug they gave me when I had the port put in. I said "Maybe I should have had general anesthetic for this…" Dr. Chow kind of chuckled, but not in a bad way… I didn't call the drug the "IDGAS" drug to her, but she knew exactly what I meant. At least 4 more times in slightly different locations, I yelped with the pain. Each time she was astonished, but thankfully, immediately injected me with more and more anesthetic. In my mind, I was reverently thanking the person who invented anesthetic, way back when. I made a mental note to myself to "Google" it, to find out who this God was, and thank him or her! I don't know how many stitches there were, but it felt like at least 15 or more. Finally it was done! I had been on the table for almost an hour.

After my experience with relying on home care for my port installation, Dr. Chow asked me if I would prefer to do my own wound care and bandage changing. I said I could and would do it myself. She asked me if we had medical supplies at home. I said all I needed would be the waterproof coverings to use in the shower. Nurse Emily lowered the table and let me get dressed, and handed me just a few waterproof bandages. I thought that was a bit stingy, but perhaps that is all I will really need.

Before I left, I asked Dr. Chow if there would be pain afterward, once all the freezing came out, she replied, "Well normally there isn't pain but with you there could be." Great, I thought. Wayne & I walked out of the Henderson and I commented that I was glad I was wearing soft soled shoes (Nike freestyle, slipper-like running shoes) as each step was again painful. Before we even got next door at the Juravinski, I was in a lot of pain. He suggested I wait at Juravinski & he would go & get the car to pick me up there. I agreed. I felt every bump in the road on the way home. It was brutal! As soon as I got home I took 2 oxycodene pills and went to lie down. I started to feel dizzy from the drugs within 15 minutes so I went to bed and slept for over 4 hours.

I told Dr. Chow, "I am not a text-book case." She agreed.

Medically Induced Menopause

All the things I was prepared for, the treatments, the symptoms, the drugs and the side effects, etc. I was NOT prepared for medically induced menopause. No one mentioned that this might be a side effect of the treatment. I was well prepared for chemotherapy and I even had to go to chemo class before my first treatment. Strange, no one mentioned menopause. No one mentioned attending a menopause class. I had heard about hot flashes but had never experienced them, of course! I never knew about reduced libido or how that feels. I didn't know about the dryness…down there…luckily I didn't experience the mood swings, or the depression but I think that is just because the cancer treatments already kicked the snot out of me, so I have nothing left for my moods to swing from!

Sudden onset of menopause happens abruptly! One minute you are your happy little self and the next minute you feel that you are suddenly on the verge of spontaneous combustion! With regular onset of menopause, things happen gradually, with time for your body and mind to adjust to each change – the hot flashes, the forgetfulness, the night sweats, the brain fog, the vaginal dryness, etc.etc. (I know I haven't listed all the "pleasures" of menopause, but I wanted to leave a few for you to be surprises later on!) Medically induced menopause is like getting hit by a truck. BAM! You're in a hot flash quicker than you can "Shut the FRONT DOOR!" and what the hell was that anyway?! Are you SURE I was not abducted by aliens and they messed around with my lady bits and now I'm all messed up! Meonpause definitely comes under my title of "Other Freaky Stuff"!

Symptoms that persist
March 4, 2010

Tearing of my eyes - periodically
Nose dripping
Toe nails falling off and cracking half way up – ouch!
Aches & pains in my joints
Mobility in my right arm & shoulder has decreased again
Port site – still irritating, itchy, little stabs of pain periodically, hurts to touch

Menopause
Dry skin, vaginal dryness
My eyelids have less elasticity and more dryness & irritation
My skin has aged considerably!
Knees & ankles that crackle like a campfire
Weight gain
Lack of energy & stamina & strength

Oh sure, and of all the cancers out there, and I have to get the one that is most likely to make you gain weight! Gotta love that too!

It seems to me that we have made a lot of progress in the treatment of cancer. We may or may not have a cure and there is lots of controversy about this, but in the meantime, I choose to be grateful for what we have made better! You typically think about a cancer patient who is bald headed, gaunt, dragging his or her butt around due to lack of energy. With the research and testing, I can honestly tell you that during my treatment for breast cancer, I never puked once. Sure I felt nauseous, but I never actually upchucked! Yes, I'm pretty proud of that!

What I have learned is that there are so many different types of cancer and even within breast cancer, there are so many differences that every cancer case is individual and therefore the treatments will vary. In addition to the different treatments, there are different side effects and everyone reacts differently as well. Some people end up with significant chronic pain, and others with peripheral neuropathy – little to no feeling in the extremities, toes and fingers and other small parts of the body, which are rich in nerve endings. Think about that one...

There are a lot of freaky things that suddenly become normal for you, once you find out you have cancer!

"If you see someone without a smile, give them one of yours!"

5 Hope, Kindness & Inspiration

May 12, 2009

Great things about having Breast Cancer:

You can surround yourself in pink everything, & not one person complains!
My house smells like a beautiful & fragrant flower garden!
I have more fresh flowers in my house now, than I ever could have imagined and I love every single beautiful bloom! And the biggest plus is I'm ALIVE to enjoy them!! (They're on my dining room table, not beside my casket!)
You can go to the mail box and get some nice cards instead of all bills.
Friends MAKE SURE they find time to see you!
It's okay to cry – in fact, it's encouraged.
You get lots of hugs!
I get to savour my hubby's and my friend's delicious cooking, instead of my own crappy cooking.
No one expects me to exercise, in fact people encourage me not to do too much!
I can sleep in all I want and it's regarded as listening to my body's needs, not being lazy.
When you finally do get outside for a little walk, everything smells super amazing ~ even way better than you remembered it!
You can leave your tea or water cup down where ever you left it and not feel too guilty.
You can NOT unload the dishwasher and not feel too guilty.
Sunshine feels even more Heavenly than it always did before!
I get a break from being Mom's Taxi.

I really know who my girlfriends & friends are! I'm so lucky!
I get to see the best in people!
I get spoiled ~ big time!
I have a great excuse to dress for comfort!
No treats are taboo!
I have the luxury of more time for reading & writing!
I am a lot less concerned & self conscious about my c-section scar, because it pales in comparison to my brand new breast surgery scar!
I will save money on shaving cream, razor blades, eye brow waxing & brazillian waxings!
People will really have to love me for my inner beauty because I know now, it won't be because of my "nice" tits!
No one expects me to wear a bra! Yeah!

Awkwardness & funny things people say

I am grateful that I got a "popular" kind of cancer, if I had to get cancer. No one ever makes jokes about prostrate or lung cancer, but everyone loves to talk about boobs! Everyone loves boobs. I love to talk about boobs! Still, it's often amusing what comments people make and what questions they ask. Sometimes I say I donated that breast to science. People don't always clue in to that right away. They just give me a funny, questioning look. I want to get the t-shirt that says, "Of course they're fake. My real ones tried to kill me." Or the t-shirt that says, "If they have to be fake they might as well be fabulous."

I've had someone ask me, "Well, where is it?" (referring to the cancer-filled breast that was cut off...to which I absently replied, "in the hospital, in a lab... hopefully not on e-Bay!")
Which one is it? I can't tell! (...and you need to know this because...)
Will you get implants? How big will you go? Don't go too big!
Do you want to use some of my fat?

How soon can you have reconstructive surgery?

Will you wake up with tits? (They better be tits and not testicals!)

Can I come with you to *shop* for your new boobies? (Shop?! Really?!)

How do you pick the size? (Sears catalogue, of course, in the back of the Bra Section!)

Will your new boobs feel like boobs? (Will you want to feel them to judge for yourself?)

Can I see them once you get them? (...of course!)

What do you mean you won't have nipples.

Where are your nipples? (damn good question!)

Hey, you will look like Barbie! (I don't think so, but you can dream!)

Are you going to lose your hair? You will look good bald!

I've experienced both bold and bashful comments and questions. One evening, when going out to a party, for laughs I wore a little card pinned to my chest with a tiny pink ribbon, where my boob used to be, and it read, "*Sorry, closed for renovation.*" One of the men I ran into that evening was so conscious of trying NOT to look at my chest, that he was not even able to make eye contact with me when we spoke. He was so embarrassed that he kept looking well over my head. I almost had to jump up to try to meet his eyes as he spoke to me. It was as if his inner voice kept telling him, "Don't look at her chest! Don't look at her chest!!!! Don't look at her chest!!!!" I found that rather hilarious!

I have also come up with a few names for *my girls* while they are under "renovation/reconstruction"!

"Boob Rocks" – because with the tissue expander in, they are as hard as rocks, and I hope they will eventually become "Boobs that rock"!.

"Franken-tits" – not unlike Frankenstein, they have been stitched together and bear the scars

"Tattered Ta-tas"

"Foobs" – fake boobs, a term I did not invent but found on YSC website (Young Survivor Coalition)

Gifts that Come from Adversity

Pink Day at my School, Sherwood Secondary, Hamilton, Ontario

A couple of the teachers, Kathy Morris and Vesna Pankerichan, and I'm not sure who else, took it upon themselves to organize a "Pink Day" at the high school where I teach. Kathy asked me if I would mind, if they did this in my honour and to promote breast cancer awareness, and I was very touched by the idea. When the day came, I was recovering from my first mastectomy and hadn't started my chemotherapy treatments yet, so I was just sitting at home when the first email of photos came in from "Pink Day"! There was a photo of the Principal, Vice Principals and a few Admin staff and teachers and a few students, standing in the front foyer, holding a large hand painted banner, which ready, "Get Well Soon Mrs. Schreuer." It was pretty and decorated with painted pink flowers! Not only that, everyone was wearing pink! I was very touched! Tears started flowing and immediately I thought, "What the heck am I doing here at home? I need to be at school!" That is the least I can do is be there when they are going to all this to support me and make me feel loved! I have always felt that Sherwood is like a second family to me and this certainly confirmed that! I couldn't believe it! I grabbed my pink t-shirt that says "Save the ta-tas!" and drove over to Sherwood to see what was happening and show them how much I appreciate all the kindness and support! I was so touched by all the random acts of kindness! Brenda Nicholls the Health Care, and Esthetics teacher, organized free, pink nail painting and pink ribbon face painting in the foyer, for anyone who wanted to take part. Some of the boys even chose to have their nails painted pink! Lots of students and teachers had pink ribbons painted on their cheeks and one of the teachers, Gary Deveau, had them paint a pink ribbon on the top of his bald head! What a sport! So many students wore pink! Sherwood spirit was alive! Nearly everyone sported something pink, somewhere that day! Some of the male teachers wore pink ties or pink shirts! Some people wore pink underwear! I just took their word on that! There was every shade of pink I could imagine. All the staff and every student got into the spirit! It was completely heartwarming! Some students wore pink wigs! It was a crazy pink day! Another teacher, who is the Advisor for our Yearbook, organized for the entire school to go out on the field behind the school and get a group photo done! It was amazing to see all those students and staff wearing pink!

Kathy made me a beautiful album of photos from the day and gave it to me! Dawn Sawford had some peer helper students in her class paint the sign and it was beautiful! It brought tears to my eyes! Brenda also made a slide show of the day and emailed it to me! A few people emailed me photos of the day too! Even students I didn't teach got into the spirit of pink. Conversations were heard that you would never expect to hear among teenagers, especially teen-age boys. They were overheard talking about the importance of breast cancer awareness. "Yeah, we gotta save those boobies!"

Some of the teaching staff commented on the different atmosphere that they experienced in the school that day. Many teachers reported an overwhelming kindness and gentleness that is not always present. Any rough edges or pressing problems seemed to take the day off too. The Pink theme and the promotion of breast cancer awareness permeated the entire school atmosphere and it seemed to have a calming effect on everyone!

Ultimately, I felt incredibly touched and supported in my journey. It made me feel boosted up and supported to take on the next grueling part of what was coming for my treatments – the dreaded chemotherapy. For the day, my worries and insecurities were lightened and as my school community came together for me and for all those affected by breast cancer, I felt the comfort of their love and concern and I did not feel so alone in what I was about to face! I am so grateful to everyone who organized and participated in this. I often look back on my Pink Day album, because it brings me such a warm, comforted feeling. It was really special! I love my Sherwood Family!

Lobsterfest

Each year we get a group of friends together and attend the Annual Ancaster Lobsterfest! It's a great event and all proceeds go to local charities. The table who wins for the best theme, costumes, etc. gets a prize of $500 to donate to the charity of your choice!

In May 2009, our friends Michele and Alan thought an excellent theme for our group would be "Breast Cancer Awareness"! Michele & Alan organized everything! We didn't even know about everything that they were planning, until the evening came! Michele had purchased pink t-shirts for all the ladies which read, "Save the ta-ta's!" For the men in our group, she had purchased white t-shirts that read, "Real Men Wear Pink"! Alan wore pink shorts, which got him a lot of attention! They even had shirts made for our children and they both said, "I Wear Pink for my Mom" , with a picture of us on the back.

Every shirt had the pink ribbon on it and on the back of each shirt they had screen printed a photo of me with that person and a funny bi-line! Each shirt had "Team Carolyn" on the back except mine, which has "My Team"! We were surprised and thrilled to have these shirts to wear to the party! I was feeling a little tentative about the Lobsterfest, since I had just had my mastectomy barely 3 weeks before. I was concerned about having the energy and stamina, but we were so psyched, it all turned out fabulous!

Some of the T-shirt's read:

Alan's:	"Hey Cancer, my friend Carolyn's going to kick your ass!"
Michele's:	"Save a tittie, cop a feel!"
Wayne's:	"I wear pink for my wife."
Mine:	"Pardon my appearance while I'm under reconstruction!"
Colleen:	"Breast friends"
Kim:	"Breast friends"
Don:	"I do free breast exams."
Gary:	"Squeeze a boob, save a life."

It was absolutely awesome!

Because I didn't want anyone to feel uncomfortable, and I wanted to sort of break the ice, I made a little sign and pinned it to my chest where my right breast used to live. It read "Sorry, closed for renovation." And I pinned it on with a pink ribbon pin.

Wayne got bright pink, Fox40 breast cancer whistles from Ron Foxcroft for everyone. We got pink leis and pink BC lanyards, pink scarves tied here and there and a giant helium filled pink ribbon balloon over three feet tall, which we secured to our table! We had a pink ribbon umbrella too! Michele & Alan also ordered a bunch of pink, breast cancer support wrist bands and we all had some. Someone decided to sell some to anyone who wanted one, and a lot of people wanted one! They sold them for $5 each and we made about $200 which I took to Juravinski Cancer Centre! We enjoyed the lobster dinner, we really enjoyed the dancing and each other but most of all we enjoyed the connection with so many people who came up to us and applauded, supported, sympathized and many of whom were also touched by cancer! It was amazing and enlightening! We didn't win the $500 prize for our theme, but it didn't matter! We had a fabulous time and we did our part to raise some money and awareness for breast cancer! It was a great night!

Saints: In My Humble Opinion

I was sitting in church with my daughter and received a wonderfully naughty text from a friend when I started thinking about my relationship with God and how my Catholic faith was working for me, or how I was functioning within its confines. Our daughter's sacrament of Confirmation is coming up and she offered to help distribute little cards with a picture of a new – recently appointed "Saint" – Andre Bessette or something like that. I picked up the little card, no so unlike a baseball or hockey card, only a bit smaller & thinner. I looked at the picture of some old dude sporting a stiff (easy now…) …collar, what the Catholic church obviously deems respectable.

My friend beside me whispered, "This may be cynical but, do you ever wonder when you see these guys, if they are some of the ones who have done "things" to boys! That hadn't crossed my mind until then, but what did come to my mind was why should this dude get his little hockey card pic and pseudo bio of his soft skills printed and distributed to our church and who knows where else. "Saint Andre … spoke with intensity… inspired hope in everyone who met him." Hey, I want to be like that! "He gave people common-sense advice and was able to empathize with those he counseled… his warm sense of humour drew people to him… and inspiration to us,, gave (his) life selflessly and never abandoned those who turned to (him)." Sounds like a pretty nice fella, eh! I want to be totally like that and at the risk of sounding conceited, I would say that if you asked my friends, they would say most of those things about me. The priest called the Saint card, a little "gift". Hmmm… don't go there! I try constantly to reign in my filthy mind, but it seldom works and sometimes it

82

just requires more energy than I am willing to part with! How many other things have priests called, "little gifts"?! Ugh! Really don't go there! I turned the card over to read the "accomplishments" of this dead man. I thought, not so unlike a lot of wonderful people I know, really.

What got my head spinning (not as in needing an exorcist kind of way – just inside, for now anyway!) was just how many wonderful people I know who I would deem Saints. Friends, Family, Angels, Colleagues, Strangers... call them what you want, but in my opinion, I could research, produce & print up cards of my Saints! Only thing is I would have my female Saints wearing lovely soft feather boas because they are a lot more fun and feminine than a stiff white collar and an ankle length robe over pants.

I was talking to my friend Susan in Hammonds Plains, Nova Scotia and she, for one, could be a Saint. Susan is always incredibly modest and I embarrass her by telling her how wonderful she is and I try not to put her on a pedestal, but it's hard for me because I admire Susan so much!

I could seriously, very easily do a Saint card for my "Saint Susan". Come to think of it, I am fortunate to have the comfort & strength of many Saint friends! Saint Colleen, Saint Michele, Saint Vesna, Saint Beth, Saint Megg, Saint Lisa...

After all, it's just a picture of someone in an extremely non-revealing outfit, and on the back, a paragraph about their "soft skills" and perhaps a notion about their E.Q.

I wonder what the reaction will be when I start publishing my own pack of Saint cards?! I think it will be fun!

"Life is not about waiting for the storms to pass. It's about learning how to dance in the rain."

83

6 Hospital "Culture"

"It's not the size of the dog in the fight, it's the size of the fight in the dog."

Pre-Op – Hey, it's all New to Me!

When I was spending the day doing pre-op stuff, a lot of things struck me. Because I had breast cancer, there wasn't any pain. It's odd to feel like the healthiest person in a room waiting your turn for surgery and going through all the motions to suddenly become a sick person. For one thing, I was totally unprepared for how much time this process would take. It basically took all day! I had to have a blood test – that wasn't hard. Then I went to another area of the hospital to check in. Wait. Read. Chat. Try to remain calm. Try not to think about the inevitable tomorrow. Wait. Try to be patient.

I had to have an ECG. I had to do this topless, which I thought was kind of weird. No sheet or anything but it was a very quick procedure, although you never know that once you get started. There was not even a hint of modesty, but it didn't bother me. Tomorrow I would be losing a breast, so what the heck if some nurse or technician should see me laying there topless, with the same interest level as if they were looking at a wall.

She hooked up electrodes with very sticky tabs on me in a variety of places. The ECG took about a minute or two, if that. It was painless and she got a print out of what my heart rhythm was like, from what I could tell. I asked her if everything looked normal (whatever normal is!) and she said yes. She peeled off the printout with a satisfied rip. She peeled off the electrodes and I

84

asked if that was all. She said yes, and I got dressed. Great, I thought, that was easy. I wandered back down the hall to see Wayne, feeling good that we only had 2 more things to "accomplish" for pre-op.

In the meantime, in the waiting room, I noticed a basket of knitting. I was tired of looking at magazines and pretending I was interested in reading my book, so I picked up the basket and wondered if I remembered how to knit. I had learned in brownies back when I was probably about 7 or 8. I had barley knit since. Sure enough I remembered how! It was a novel way to pass the time and I read the card inside the basket. Each square knitted would be eventually sewn together to make a blanket for someone who was ill, so I thought that was very nice.

Meanwhile, we were getting hungry. The day was passing. We spoke to the receptionist to see if we could go grab a bite to eat and she assured us that we had time. Everyone is the waiting room was significantly older than me. I couldn't help but think that they were looking at me as a fraud, with no reason to be in pre-op, looking like the picture of health. Almost everyone in the waiting room was waiting for hip or knee replacements, so they were visibly in pain. It kind of made me feel good in a way, to seem like the healthy one.

When someone dropped a magazine under the chair. I leapt to retrieve it for them. When a woman lost her glasses, I felt it was my quest, the hunt them down for her. I would be the legs and speed of dismal "Pre-Op" ship.

I would be the helper, so I wouldn't have to think about my pending misery and degradation. I could focus on my "room-mates" and be their healthy & helpful assistant. After all, I was the most mobile "sick person" in the room. Silly things that amuse me, while trying to create a diversion in my own thoughts...

Of course, there was a lot more waiting and we realized that we would not be finished in time to pick up our daughter from school at 3:40. Wayne made some phone calls to arrange for her to go to a friend's house, and we waited. Finally we got to see a nurse who went over a huge checklist with me about dos & don't s. She asked me if I had questions. The only question I felt burning was, "Can this really be happening to me?" I liked to fantasize that I would wake up and it would all have been a very vivid, but completely false, bad dream.

I told the nurse I didn't' have any questions, even though some of her questions brought tears to my eyes. She told me to pick out a croissant shaped pillow from the shelves behind me. I picked out the brightest colour that caught my eye – red, and took it gratefully, even though I had no idea whatsoever, whatever I would use it for. She likely told me, but like so many conversations, parts were a blur. Something to do with breast cancer... I felt a little numb and Wayne & I left that office and were back in the waiting room once again. We now only needed to meet with the anestitist, as our final step of Pre-Op.

The enthusiasm I felt for knitting and the cause that the knitting represented, was no longer a spark inside me. The waiting game had me feeling worn out. Eventually by about 4:00, the nurses and receptionist had gone and there were only a few couples left waiting to see the anestitist. I realized that we would be last.

We had our turn and it was very straightforward. This doctor just went over a checklist with me about meds and what to take and not to eat or drink past 9am, etc. It was all very common sense. We waited all day for this? Basically, the important thing was to sign a consent form. Very anti-climactic really, but I would have enough to be climactic in the next few days.

The Hospital

I've noticed that hospitals LOVE rules, BUT LOVE does not rule hospitals!

Some people are familiar with hospitals, and their unique routines and "culture", from either having been a patient or having had a relative who was a patient, or perhaps they've had some kind of medical & hospital experience, etc. None of those experiences were in my background. My only experience was having a miscarriage and giving birth to my two children. It has only been in the past five years that I have even managed to overcome my hospital phobia, through my work, seeing my students at their coop placements in hospitals. If I sound naïve, about my expectations and observations, that is why.

Post Surgery & My Roomies!

Good thing I have semi-private coverage and I was willing to pay for a private room! Ha! Ha! It made no difference whatsoever! Because there weren't any beds available, I was sent to a ward room on the 5th floor, already inhabited with 3 men! I already felt vulnerable and uncomfortable emotionally and otherwise. This was the icing on the cake!

As I was being wheeled into the room, I heard a nurse telling off an 87 year old man from Montreal, who wanted to be naked. She was giving him a serious tongue lashing! I heard her say, "We have a young lady coming in here! You need to get your clothes on and keep them on! Stop taking them off! She does NOT want to see you naked!" etc.

Mr. Naked Montreal was in the bed next to me. It did cross my mind about what he might do, if he wandered over to me and would he have any ideas, if he was naked with a "young lady" even a single breasted one, in the room with him. I gave myself a pep talk about not thinking I was "all that" and who would be interested in me in any kind of sexual way, in my current condition, but part of my brain still worried and I felt vulnerable and afraid!

My roommate directly across from me was comatose and seemed to be completely hooked up to tubes and wires. Clearly he was not going anywhere. He looked like he was in pretty dire shape. I saw a man probably around my age at his bedside earlier in the day, trying desperately to talk to him. He pleaded, "Dad... Dad?... Dad!!!???" "Dad, wake up!"...but no response came from the tubed man lying in the bed. It was heart-breaking, as I couldn't help but notice the younger man at his bedside, hold his Dad's hand and then hang his head down in despair. I empathically felt the desolate wave of heartache wash over to my side of the room!

My roomie diagonally across from me was about 67, a sweet fellow with a darling attentive wife. He was spending his last night in the hospital and was going home the next day, so he and his wife were very happy! The day following my second surgery, I was able to get up and get him some ice water a couple of times, so I felt good about that.

So much for a private room! There was nothing private about that experience.

Call button – all tied up! Help me please!
(Cue Beach Boys, song "Help, help me Rhonda!")

After my second surgery in two days, I awoke in the darkness of some unknown hour I classified in my brain as the "middle of the night". Surprisingly I slept soundly through the noise and chaos of the 5th floor, and someone incessantly moaning "Help me!" down the hall! Drugs will do that for you! What woke me was the overwhelming realization that I needed to go pee. It seems to be the basic necessities and basic human dignities that are difficult to handle in a hospital.

Once my head began to clear and my mind raced to the present, I realized that my nightmare was still an ugly reality. I was still stuffed with tubes, still in a hospital and still barely able to move. I had oxygen tubes in my nose for breathing, the IV and all stuck mid way up my left arm and my right arm was incapacitated by the surgery. Also on my right side were the two JP drains on tubes sticking out of me. I bet Robo Cop never looked this attractive. Ha!

Amazingly amidst all the tubes & wires, I managed to find the call button to ask for help from the nurse. It was still loosely wrapped in my right hand where the nurse had placed it as I fell asleep. At first I tried to sit up & it was at that attempt that I realized that my gorgeous hospital gown was not snapped across my shoulders. It immediately slid down my body leaving my scary surgical area one still intact breast, exposed.

Luckily I had the extreme privacy of a loosely drawn curtain on one side, and I was only open to the front, the area I was facing! The man in the bed directly across from me was sadly comatose, being even more encumbered than me with his breathing tubes, etc. No worries of him coming to, and if he did, it might have been a very good thing for him, poor guy.

I removed the oxygen tubes from my nose and tried to find a place to leave those tubes untangled from me so I could plan my escape to pee. It was no use! I had to face it. I needed help! I just could not do this alone. I pressed the call button and waited. The nurse's voice came over the PA into the room, which I was not expecting. I was concerned for my roommates. Would they wake up? Would they be upset? I interrupted their sleep. Oh how I wished I had some privacy and the use of my pre-surgery body!!!

I attempted a response to Nurse Donna's question, "Do you need help?" My voice was hoarse, raspy and too quiet to be detected by the intercom. Of course I need help, I thought in frustration, otherwise why would I press this damn "HELP" button. I'm not some rat hoping for a food pellet to be released. Please, damn it, come and help me, I pleaded in my mind. She would have no idea that I didn't come to this decision lightly. I hate to inconvenience people and be a pain, but I really needed help! I was desperate. I wondered if I might accidentally pee in the bed before I ever managed to escape its confines. I attempted another few words to plea my case. My raspy, voice squeaked, "I need to go to the bathroom." It was all I could muster. Nothing….

OMG, did she hear me? The Nurse's voice on the other end answered me with a questioning "Hellllllooo?????" Not good. I thought I am going to have to do this alone. I continued to fumble in the dark, now nearly tearful at trying to manage and take care of such a basic need. It was so humiliating and frustrating. I thought I would try to call button one more time, just in case some one might venture down the hallway to check on me. In my mind, I tried to "will" the nurse to please come & see me.

The second attempt at the call button, evoked the same PA response. My attempts to communicate were the same – useless! Tears of frustration began to flow, and I fervently wished I was not alone. I wished for Wayne or anyone to help.

I semi laid back in bed and sighed, trying not to cry too loudly to disturb my roommates – thinking that is the last thing these 3 men need to know, in the middle of the night is that I need to go pee!

Somehow I managed to escape the confines of my bed and the binding tubes & wires. I slid down to the floor and reached the bathroom door, pulling along my IV pole, trying not to get it trapped in the door. As I stepped into the bathroom, I realized I was standing in a puddle of pee – not mine! As grossed out as I was, I stood on one leg and reached for a towel to cover the floor so I could get to the toilet without having to completely wade through the yellow puddle. As I was standing there perched like a sad Flamingo on one leg, nurse Donna showed up at the bathroom door.

A beam of light reached into the room and she was a welcomed silhouette in the doorway, as a look of mystified horror came over her face and she exclaimed, "OH MY GOD!". I had no idea what was wrong and expected the worst – something I hadn't noticed – perhaps an open wound seething somewhere on my body, that she could see but I couldn't?! Yikes! I asked, "What's wrong?!"

She seemed much more concerned now, than the voice had indicated through the PA. She gasped astonishingly, and I braced myself for more bad news of something devastating, that I had not yet noticed. "You're standing on one leg!" she exclaimed! I apologetically explained, "There's pee on the floor. I'm trying not to step in it." I told her I needed to get up to go pee. I apologized. I couldn't do it by myself. She explained, to my relief, that she had never seen anyone stand on one leg after just having surgery! I didn't have any open, seething wounds after all! Phew!

She quickly & efficiently wrapped the IV wires around so I could move with it, and helped me in the washroom and then back to bed, thank goodness. Phew, what a relief. Thank goodness that ordeal was over for now. She asked me about the pain and then she topped up my meds in the IV and I welcomed the sleep that followed again.

What is Vegetarian?

What is vegetarian? Does meatloaf with gravy qualify? Yuck! Although I was grateful for food while in the hospital, it never ceased to amaze me how unhealthy and unappetizing the food actually was! Yikes! Sometimes, I wondered how anyone could get better on such unhealthy choices. It also surprised me when someone brought in a dinner for me, which consisted of meatloaf and various other non-descript "food" items. I asked, meekly, do you know if it's vegetarian, just before uncovering the "treasure" under the stainless steel lid. The person delivering said, if that is what you asked for, then it must be. When I lifted the lid, I was greeted by a small mound of pale mashed potatoes, a pinch of grayish green peas, and a hunk of meatloaf, all doused somewhat generously in a sand coloured gravy. Ick! Having been vegetarian for almost 3 decades, I was not impressed. I gently explained to the kind dinner delivery person that this was definitely NOT vegetarian and asked if I could please have something else – non meat. Of course, I don't do gravy either, so I couldn't even eat the peas or potatoes. Although I don't think I was missing out on much by not being able to eat the vegetables. I would have to wait a while for something else, but it had to be better than this!

More Blood?

Sometimes I think some of the vampire cast from Twilight, were hanging out in the nooks and crannies of the hospital. It seemed to me that every time I was woken up, someone wanted to take blood from me! It got to be quite creepy, and so many times I had to remind them not to use my right arm where I had most of my lymph nodes removed. I didn't want to risk getting lymphadema on top of all the other stuff I had to deal with! I wanted to put a sign or perhaps Caution tape around that arm, so they would get the message! They were having a hard time getting blood from me, so I asked if they could possibly take it from the I.V. that was already stuck in my left arm. Well, that was a bit of a fiasco too. I could see the blood leaking from this place on an ongoing basis, so what was the big deal, I thought.

One particularly rough male nurse came in to take blood. I was getting fed up. I asked him what this blood was needed for. He had no idea. He just rudely began slapping my right hand looking for a vein and I was barely awake. I snapped awake to ask him just what he thought he was doing. Perhaps he always does this to comatose patients and was not used to the patient coming to, and questioning him. It took a bit of convincing but finally he left my right hand and arm alone and with my pleading, he called for the I.V. nurse to come and take the blood from my I.V. I figured I already had the pain and nuisance of having an I.V. stuck in my arm, they might as well use the darn thing.

After 2 surgeries in 2 days, my mastectomy and my hematoma, I was now officially on my road to recovery. I had been in the hospital for 3 days and was itching to escape. It was noisy and stuffy and impersonal and I always felt so incredibly vulnerable and at the mercy of everyone there.

The only time I felt a bit secure was when my doctor was in my room, talking to me, and when my husband was there with me. What I did find though, was that time flies when you're having fun, but it also flies when you're not doing anything!

Thankfully, I got home on Saturday, the day before Mother's Day and on Mother's Day, as painful as it was, at least I got to wake up in my own bed and be with my family. It felt so good to be home! At least most of the psychological trauma was over. Now there was just the physical to deal with and I felt ready to face that!

Home care Nurses were booked to come and change my dressings and make sure I knew how to empty the 2 JP drains that were installed in my chest, where my breast used to live. I was taught how to "milk" the drains and measure the output and all kinds of other gross stuff, but after almost 3 weeks of no showering (Easy now, no need to hold your nose....only baths) Seventeen days since surgery, I finally got the last drain pulled out and that was a huge relief.

Hospital adhesive tape ~ What the hell is that made of?

It's been 3 weeks today, May 28, since I had the surgery and would you believe that I am still finding bits of tape residue on parts of my body! I shower, I scrub, I rub & scrape what I can find and still, every day, I find a few more little pieces. Today in the shower I actually found two more pieces of adhesive that held my IV in – yikes!

Shouldn't the troops be utilizing this substance! Talk about staying power!

It reminds me of a few lines from Robin Williams, when he talks about baby poo. Yes, baby poo. He does a comedy piece where he is a new Dad and he is changing his baby's diaper and he is desperately trying to remove the baby poo from the clothing of his baby. He says something about, "What is baby poo? It seems like part Velcro and part nuclear waste!" That line reminds me of the tape they use at hospitals – part Velcro and part nuclear waste! I have since found out that not only is this stuff nearly impossible to remove but to make matters more challenging, I am allergic to it! I get a red, itchy and later painful rash if the adhesive tape is left on my skin for an hour or more! Great!

As much as I admire hospital staff, nurses, doctors, technicians, etc. I realize I never want to be one of them!

Rules designed to facilitate, I will honour. Rules designed to impede, I will overcome.

7 Chemotherapy

"Change is always difficult."

Chemotherapy Treatment ~ How does it feel?

Well, I had my first chemo treatment on Friday June 26, 2009and today marks day 4, post first treatment. Today I do not feel good. I took myself to the hospital for some blood work to be done before the port can be installed on Friday, July 3, Wes' 14 th birthday. I went to Juravinski with the efficiency that, I imagine, a ghost travels the Earth. I felt like I floated. I couldn't eat this morning. I didn't even have my usual cup of tea. Even water was not appetizing. I was hoping for a bit of appetite but nothing.

I felt like I floated past everyone, every soul, and I could barely make out any faces. I spoke to someone on the phone at Hurst Place to make an appointment and the words that fell out of my mouth felt like someone's else's words. It was like an out of body experience. My back and neck feel like someone went half a centimeter under my skin everywhere and bruised every inch. Even the water from the shower hurt when it hit my skin on my shoulders, neck and back. I had the blood test. For some reason I felt weepy. I contemplated going to sit out on the mountain brow in a brief interlude from the rain, and crying. I wondered if I was indulging myself feeling sorry for myself, but then I thought of Victoria home alone and feeling sick and I decided to come straight home instead. Sitting hurts, lying down hurts, and when standing – my legs feel shaky. I noticed how easy it is to see my ears now, through my hair. I am losing hair – not in clumps yet, but I can tell. My stomach feels very tender and queasy. I don't feel nauseous but I do feel icky. It's like a constant never ending toxic pain across my front waistline.

I am sick of hospitals already. That is not a good sign. I've only just begun! No position feels comfortable. No activity seems desirable. No food seems to entice me. It's an effort to read. I feel lonely but I'm too lacking in ambition to call someone and talk and besides, I don't want to bring anyone down because there is nothing anyone can do to help me. I feel like I am barely hanging on and the very scary thing is that this is jut the beginning! What will I do?!

Janet McNulty phoned today and that cheered me up! Although I did break down a little. I think she was okay with that. I got a lovely sweet card from Susan Flewelling which really touched my heart too. Susan wants to come & visit me. Barb Fraser called me too, so really it is a good day but I still feel like crap. It helped. Even sitting here to write a mere 300-500 words is causing me so much pain in my back muscles. I need air but I can't carry myself outside.

How do I feel? I feel like there is something foreign and toxic in my belly, needing to get out. I need to have a "BM" (bowel movement), but last night I didn't feel like taking the "Senocot" (a natural laxative to help get things moving down there). I just wanted a break from drugs. I feel so icky! It's like I have a brain fog. I can't get interested in anything. It's just such a gross feeling.

"When she was good she was really, really good, but when she was bad she was horrid…" (Little Miss Muffet, Mother Goose)

This is not for the faint of heart. If you are squeamish about bodily functions (or malfunctions!) skip the next part. You've been warned!
July 29, 2009

How about the "horrid"? How do I feel? Well, let me pour it out – As I have probably said before, my body feels like a toxic waste dump in the days after my chemo treatments. Yes, I can say it feels flu-ish, although I fortunately am not one to get the flu – hardly ever so I can only imagine... I feel generally very unwell. My heart races when I move at all, even to walk up the stairs, I feel I will nearly pass out. I see black around my vision, but then it comes back. My digestive system is no longer a pleasure tube or a well-oiled machine that serves me. My head aches in different spots. I feel pain even when the water from the shower touches my head, my neck, my shoulders, my chest where my breast used to be. The shower used to be a pleasure and now it too, is painful. The back of my neck and my lower back are carrying a lot of tension and ache in every position. My mouth is cut open at the corners and it stings when I open it or yawn, or anything. I have the mouth ulcers, of course. They sting and they bother me all the time – but what can I do? I am keeping up with the disgusting rinse of baking soda & salt. It helps a bit, even though it tastes disgusting!

There are cracks at the sides of my mouth, that hurt when I yawn or open my mouth. They sting and they are not healing. Even though I am rinsing my mouth out, the cracks are not getting any better. I put "polysporin" on the corners, and Vaseline, but still, it persists. *TMI Warning*! Keeping my bowels moving has never been a chore for me but it sure is now. I reluctantly force stool softners down my throat and hope for the best. Now every BM (bowel movement) is painful and there is blood. My butt bleeds from passing everything. That can't be good! I guess I have hemorrhoids. Ick! I can tell you for sure it hurts like hell. Even after I apply the "Annusol", my butt hole burns & burns. I have what I assume to be acid reflux, where it feels like there is always something wanting to come up your throat. No amount of swallowing will take it back down. I am hungry but I can't think of a single thing I am remotely interested in eating. I am thirsty but even my usual pleasures offer me no comfort at all. I used to enjoy & look forward to a cup of tea and or a nice cold glass of water – not now. I can barely be bothered. Eating at all is an effort to fill a gap. Drinking is an effort. I don't feel like any food or drink is celebratory. Nothing seems remotely desirable. Now my taste buds are changing and I seem to notice more texture than flavour. I just look at the medicine bottles and feel nauseous. Ick! Ick! Ick! I don't want people to tell me to feel better. I know I will and that this is just what I must do to pay my dues. It's what I must endure to ensure the cancer is killed. It's time, but it wears me down. I don't want to endure this. ... but I know I will.... There aren't any viable alternatives.

The other thing is that I am disinterested in pretty much everything. I am not interested in eating or drinking, even reading or writing. I can't think of anything to take my mind off the overwhelming feeling of "ICK!" that consumes me. Somewhere hurts all the time. I feel lethargic. Not even sleep gives me relief because my dreams are bothering me now too. I keep having a dream about a crooked, dilapidated old house, where I'm trying to live and nothing works and there are lots of problems. The floors are at an angle, the tables are at angles and things slide off and it drives me crazy! Nothing feels good or right. In the end, the floors fall through or we have to tear it down and we lose sentimental stuff. It's so devastating. I'm so sick of these dreams but I keep on having them. It's not always the same house. It's all different houses, but they all have similar problems. There is no comfort there – just problems and constant challenges and disappointment and despair! Is this my life now?

Paclitaxel – I got a new drug... What is happening to me now?

Well It's Monday and I had my first chemo cocktail of paclitaxel on Friday, my 46th birthday. It's my 5th chemo, but this is a whole new thing. Last night the pain started to hit me... I wanted to feel what it was like to some extent. I wanted to see if I could handle it. Wayne encouraged me to take Tylenol right away, as soon as we got home. I took it, but by 9:30 the pain brought tears to my eyes. I asked Victoria to get me the oxycocet and I wanted relief. Even the tips of my fingers hurt now from typing.

Pain is running down my legs, shooting across my abdomen, running through my shins like an electrical current. It stabs in my abdomen, here and there, recklessly at will. The kids want me to take them out. "Are we ready yet?" Victoria asks me. "Do you have your make up on yet? ... You don't need make up. You're beautiful", my sweet daughter tells me. I don't know if I really believe her. I know I used to but now I am feeling so battered and sexless.

I feel like a pain in Wayne's life. I can't even keep up with the house work and my parents will be here for a visit in 2 days – so much to tidy up! So many details – I wonder if I can do it at all. I feel the need to talk to someone who cares & understands, but I know I will just cry. Is it the drugs that are bringing me down? Is it me? I just don't know. I know I need to go for a walk, but I wonder how I will do with that. I wonder if I can make it and then there is the necessity for sunscreen beforehand – one more step in the process. Almost every part of me hurts! There is so much I want to take care of, but I can barely do it! It's so incredibly frustrating!

Chemo Brain

I can definitely attest to the legitimacy of "chemo fog" or "chemo brain". While I was helping my daughter Victoria gather images for her Science title page, one of the images she had printed was a microscope. What was a shocking reality for me was when I stared at this well known object, no matter how hard I concentrated, I could absolutely not come up with a word for what it is called! It seemed the harder I thought, the more entrenched the blank became. Truthfully, it scared me. I have always taken pride in my ability to communicate and my command of the English language. It took me a solid three hours before the word finally came to me! "Microscope!" How hard was that?! It floored me!

My children learned to get used to me calling the washer the toaster & the toaster the kettle. The dryer was sometimes the "white box in the mud room that doesn't wash". The phone would sometimes, in a desperate moment to retrieve the right word, be called the "ringing thing". I found myself stopping for a green light. I just hope I didn't go through any red lights. I certainly would not do that intentionally. Yikes!

Usually I pride myself in my ability to remember & use people's names! Names are really important to me! I would suddenly blurt out 2 or 3 names together and the first syllables would all be mixed up. My daughter babysits 3 adorable little sisters, Macy, Stella & Georgia. One day I was trying to say their names and it kept coming out "Sacy, Mella and I could not seem to get my brain to be able to straighten it out. I always joke about having "spoonism" (mixing up syllables in words) but I really do have this issue now.

I went to my appointment at my optometrist and walked out the door afterward, took my son shopping, stopped at Tim Horton's and then picked up my daughter from school.

It wasn't until I pulled into our driveway at home, that I suddenly realized that I completely forgot to pay the $80 cost of my eye check up! Suddenly, like the lights in my brain were turned on, I realized that I had completely forgotten to pay! Good thing I wasn't shoplifting!! Yikes!

Wes asked me on Sunday if he had gone to his vocal training lesson on Friday. I may have driven him, but I have no recollection of it whatsoever. I really think I didn't take him. Hmmm... we still don't know! Bizarre!

Breast Cancer's Negative Impact on my Life
As of October 27, 2009
I must preface this list with what I feel in my heart. I have some difficulty writing about this for two reasons. I am still feeling the effects of "chemo brain" as I just finished chemotherapy three weeks ago. I am not a person who focuses on the negative. Thankfully this is my nature. Focusing on the negative aspect of what I am forced to deal with, will not help my healing or my state of mind.

Chemo brain - My brain is not as strong as it used to be – I forget words sometimes, for things that are everyday things. (washer, toaster, microscope) I forget names sometimes and usually I am very good at this. It's always been a thing I pride myself on!) I can't seem to express myself as well, on my feet, as I used to be able to. I don't seem to be able to communicate as fluently as I used to be able to. I lose my train of thought more frequently.

Sometimes I catch myself in the middle of something, wondering where I was going and what I was going to do. I just do not feel as sharp, at all – brain fog. A lot of people laugh when I tell them this, and they tell me it's not the chemo & radiation treatments, it's my age. Well, it's funny how this deterioration developed rapidly during and after my treatments. I don't believe it is old age, but I do believe that chemo is to blame!

Vision – My vision has deteriorated over the past 3-4 months, during and post chemo. Reading printed material and reading on the computer is very difficult, especially at times when it seems my eyes cannot focus. Changing the distance between the material being read, does not seem to help. As my eyes have only a few lashes left and minimal eyebrows, each morning there is discharge and my eyes are crusty, itchy and sometimes foggy. Writing & editing on the computer is also difficult because of my deteriorated vision. Some people have this happen as a result of

101

chemo, but the doctors tell me that it usually returns, although I have met a few survivors, whose vision deteriorated and it stayed that way.

On Nov. 11, 2010 I have an appointment with the Ophthalmologist. I want her to check my eyes to ensure there isn't damage and to see if I need a stronger prescription. As it turned out, I did need a much stronger prescription after cancer. I ended up getting my first pair of invisible "tri-focal" glasses, and I am so happy to be able to see clearly again!

Fatigue

A lot of women will tell you about fatigue they experience. It is such a common complaint that it hardly seems worth mentioning, as it's a given. One thing is for sure. I can no longer do as much as I used to do. Everything takes me much longer than it used to and I need more down time to recover from everything – even simple tasks. Sometimes I walk up one flight of stairs and I am out of breath and I feel like I need to sit or lie down for a bit, to catch my breath. Simple tasks take me a lot longer than they used to. I definitely feel the inability to do everything I used to be able to do, before cancer!

Chest & arm pain
Headaches – eye strain, fatigue
Teary eyes
Physical
Mental – ability to concentrate diminished, finding the right word, thinking quickly – less ability
Emotional
Confidence
Energy & stamina
Relationship
Sex; body changes – digestive system, constipation, etc.
Fitness decline; Menopause; Self image

Wayne's Thoughts on Chemotherapy

Despite what I was going through, Wayne had to go through chemotherapy too. He had strong feelings about this too. Wayne had faith that chemotherapy would work. He saw it as a process, without any shortcuts. He told me that sometimes he felt guilty that he wasn't sick. It was a raw deal for our entire family! Friends too! Wayne admitted to feeling some resentment in his weaker moments because suddenly he had to handle all the responsibility alone. He felt he was always "ON" and everything fell on him to take care of! I have a little man doll and when you push his little chest, he speaks and his name is "Mr. Wonderful"! Wayne gave him to me ages ago and I love him! He says things like, "Oh can't your Mother stay another week?" and "Let's just cuddle tonight." "Oh I don't care about the ball game. I'd rather spend time with you!" "Why don't I pull in here and ask for directions?" etc. Wayne was feeling like the expectations he needed to live up to, far exceeded his ability. Wayne told me, "I'm not Mr. Wonderful!" That was his way of telling me that he was feeling too much pressure. It was very tough on him. He hated seeing me sick and adding the things I usually do, to his list of responsibilities, was huge.

The other thing that had an effect on Wayne during chemotherapy was the shock at the number of people on any given day, who were waiting for treatment in the chemo suite. He equated it to the airport lounge! It didn't matter which day I was there, the waiting area was always packed with people. I noticed that there was hardly ever anyone there who was even close to my age.

The other thing that impressed Wayne while I was going through chemotherapy, was how kind and efficient the staff were at Juravinski Cancer Centre! Even though we sometimes had to wait for more than 2 hours for my chemo, once we were in their care, we felt completely taken care of! Overall, going through chemo was a time when we both realized how much people cared for us! We were truly overwhelmed and blessed by everyone's unexpected kindness. Flowers and cards with lovely sentiments flooded in! Delicious meals appeared out of the blue and our whole family was so grateful for the outpouring of kindness that enveloped us during this horrible time!

What was good about Chemo?

Am I crazy? How could there be anything good about chemo? Here's the crazy truth!

When do you ever get to sit and talk with a friend, basically uninterrupted for 4 hours?

When do busy Moms get to sit back in a comfy chair and have someone bring them a glass of water or juice while you sit & read a book, while wrapped in a comfy blanket?

When do you get to sit down & be offered a cookie by a lovely, senior volunteer lady?

When does the world basically stop for you to sit down and think, reflect and contemplate your journey?

When do you get to gain insights into the lives and struggles and triumphs of so many people facing the battle of cancer?

When do you see life & death so closely linked, staring you right in the face, as your eyes connect with the souls around you in the chemo suite? When do you feel like a chosen one, somehow pulled out of the everyday rat race, to navigate a different path for a while and learn so much more than you would have never been privy to, if not for cancer and chemotherapy treatments? When do you get to experience the shivers down your neck and spine as you feel the collective energy, empathetically, in the chemo suite

– the positive and reassuring forces of the gentle nurses, and admin staff, the fears of some undergoing treatment, the tingles of those who desperately or bravely are taking chemo even though they know they are bravely facing death, just buying a bit more time, the terrified souls, floundering in the face of what stubbornly desires to be our killer, the comfort of angels in the friends, family, staff and volunteers who accompany us through this grueling time…

When do you get to lie on the couch, wrap up in a blanket and just "be"? When does music ever soothe like it does when you are grasping at any force in the universe to help you get through the next minutes, hours, days, weeks?

How could it be a privilege to witness first hand the pain of others and feel the wrath, the treatments inflict on your body?

How can this teach you what really matters in life? It does. It's a beat over the head with a baseball bat but I guess some of us have to learn the hard way. Perhaps I am one of them!

How can love taste sweeter than it already tasted and yet now I know, it does. How can you comprehend the value of your family, your friends and people, like you come to know through enduring chemo? Ah yes, cancer has taught me many things and I know there are still more to come. I am obsessed with not losing the lesson! Can you blame me?!

"Does it tire you or does it inspire you?" (Kris Carr)

This is the question I ask myself before agreeing to do something that someone else asks of me. Before cancer, being the social butterfly that I am, "Would you like to…?" my answer was almost always a resounding "Yes!", but now I have to be cautious and choosy with how I spend my precious energy and time. This questions helps me sort this out in my mind.

8 Radiation

Radiation

October 26, 2009 – Today I had my first of 25 radiation treatments. It's always good to get over the initial anxiety that comes from something unknown. No matter how prepared you try to be and how much information you gather, I always say, there is no teacher like experience. This afternoon, as I walked down an unfamiliar hallway in the Juravinski Cancer Centre, and dressed in those attractive and cozy pale blue cotton hospital gowns that ties in back, I felt like a patient again. Walking in I felt completely healthy, even though I have a way to go with recuperation. There is something about those gowns that makes me feel unwell and vulnerable.

Joyce was very nice to me, as she explained where things were and what the procedures were for this new (to me) phase of cancer treatment. Her warm smile made me feel more comfortable. When it was time to go into the treatment room, everyone I met called me by my first name. It actually caught me off guard but I liked it. They showed me the room where they would be when I was receiving the treatment in 21-E. They showed me the cameras that they would be looking at while I was in the room alone. They assured me that no one else could see me except for them. Katz – at least that is what her name sounded like, was very sweet too. I was a little nervous. They were so gentle, precise and accommodating and they seemed to anticipate my questions and worries, explaining every step. They made me feel very confident in their expertise.

Katz and Joyce told me to lie down on the metal slab, which they refer to as a bed. Katz, with a lovely British accent, instructed me to put my head on the "pretend pillow" which I thought was very funny! The "pretend pillow" is a circular shaped, very shallow indentation in the metal slab, where you need to place your head during treatment. Your arm goes up in what feels like kind of a right angle, beside your ear and for a minute or two you actually think, well this isn't too bad. Katz positioned me by telling me not to move and she pulled the sheets under me to help get me into the exact position. Today it took about 15 – 20 or more minutes but they said that the first day take s longer because they needed to take other pictures. After 15 or more minutes, your arm kind of goes to sleep and when you do get to remove it from the stirrup like resting place, it doesn't always move. My arm was kind of stuck in that position and they helped me move it back.

It is very precise. They talk to each other in numbers, coordinates, and use a hefty looking remote to move pieces of large equipment around to your sides, that is labeled "Do not irradiate." At times I felt like I was in a Star Trek scene and invisible things were happening to make me better. If Captain Piccard's voice came over the intercom, paging number one, I wouldn't have been completely surprised! An electronic humming noise happened each time the beam was on, which unnerved me at first. It was then that I was very conscious of my breathing, being careful not to take too deep of a breath as I had been instructed. Because I was so busy trying not to consciously take a deep breath, I was actually breathing in a more shallow way and kind of felt the need to breathe more deeply but I didn't, at least while I knew the radiation was on.

The hardest thing, other than the "bed" itself, was staying still. I made a huge effort not to move a muscle. It was tough, but I did it. At one point my wig was making my head itch. I tried not to focus on it. I tried to focus on mystery and science behind the working of the equipment. At another point my nose itched. I didn't dare move to scratch. I asked Joyce what would I do if I sneezed. She said, just don't move your arm. I was suddenly conscious of my fingers involuntarily moving in my right hand. and I immediately commanded them to stop! My right foot jerked once, but it wasn't when the radiation beam was on so that was okay. Yes, staying still was hard.

I do have a little bit of machine phobia, which I think comes from being claustrophobic. I was also unnerved when the huge circular part that the radiation passes through came close to me and circled around me. Katz picked up on this right away and assured me that the machine would not touch me. I felt like she read my mind. That was exactly what I was thinking and wondering about at that moment. The reassurance helped so much.

It is bizarre not to be able to wear anti-perspirant on my right underarm. I keep thinking I will be very sweaty but so far, so good. We will see what tomorrow brings.

May 21, 2009

Oh, so much to write about, where do I start? I just finished my Coop Part 3 Specialist Course from Queen's University yesterday and I am proud to say I finished everything & I got Honours! Yay me! Phew… Now time to get back to my own writing. I'm afraid it is going to be a bit disjointed so I think I will just write little sub headings as I go along. Relating my journey by each date, might not work for me. Right now I'm just feeling tired, very tired! I think I could sleep for a week. My head is killing me too, with a brutal headache!

Words that caress, comfort, sooth and inspire: My hubby, my kids, my dogs.

Things people say, which I love:

From: fronza@live.com
      Subject: RE: Getting to know Friends
      Date: May 26, 2009 9:53:27 AM GMT-04:00

Hi Carolyn, I just wanted to say don't be afraid of losing your hair…you're beautiful with or without hair........I know how you feel.....Hair is everything to a woman!!!! I'm still jealous of women with beautiful hair.....anytime you want to go shopping for some wigs, hats or sash, I'm your girl...I could use a few new items......just think of your beautiful kids and wonderful husband and all your good friends and family......and the strong wonderful woman you are....."Bald is beautiful" sending lots of love....Franca

Tell me, what is it you plan to do
with your one wild and precious life?
Mary Oliver from The Summer Day poem

Life is not just about learning how to survive the storms. It's about learning how to dance in the rain.

June 18, 2009
Met with Dr. Ronen Avram – Reconstruction
Thinking about DIEP procedure

They Can Rebuild Me!

This morning Wayne & I left before 7:30am to go to MAC to meet the surgeon who I will get to do my reconstruction. Wayne has golfed with Dr. Ronen Avram a few times now and speaks very highly of him. I already know I will like him. This is a perk in the realm of hospital visits and doctor appointments – or this is how we are looking at it. Dr. Avram doesn't start his clinic until 9 so he wants to see us at 8am to work us in beforehand. Very considerate of him, and he is the doctor. He uses another doctor's office and apologizes, which I find mildly amusing. He is very cute and soft spoken but seems very keen and efficient too. His second baby is due on Halloween. Ronen asks me for the update to what has transpired so far. I give his the short version and he begins to tell us about options for reconstruction. He plugs in his laptop to show us a slide show he uses for other docs in the field. We follow along. I am interested in the DIEP procedure where they take fat cells and tissue from my abdomen to transplant to make a breast mound. It would leave me with a scar across my entire hip line about where my c-section scar is. It would essentially give me a tummy tuck and would enable me to have my own flesh in my breast as opposed to having something foreign inside me like an implant. I think this is a good idea but the recovery seems difficult and so I really want another scar? How much more scaring will this take? A later procedure will construct a nipple. I am thinking about the timing. I am both encouraged and discouraged. Yes, of course, I want to eventually look "normal" but how long will all of this take? The time frame, I ask about... Could it possibly be done in December? I tell Dr. Avram I would like it to be done in December – my goal. Dr. Avram tells us that it is ultimately up to Dr. Arnold to give the go-ahead for me to have the reconstructive surgery. At this point I am accepting & respectful of his expertise and his position.

Later I consider implants too as they seem less invasive and perhaps more attractive – I don't know. But what about my left breast? More to think about ...

"My new mantra – "If they're going to be fake the might as well be fabulous!"

I saw a t-shirt on the American Breast Cancer website that said, "Of course they're fake! My first ones almost killed me!" I might have to get that shirt.

June 24, 2009
Feeling agitated tonight. It's hot & I think the air con is not working! It's 89F in our bedroom. Ick! I had the abdominal ultrasound this morning and the chest x-ray.

Tom Marsh – my former student is the x-ray technician "Now you can teach me Tom!"

So much, so little energy, so overwhelming
June 30, 2009

Look Good, Feel Better Workshop

Losing my Hair
July 11, 2009

My hair is coming out like crazy now. Wes just brushed my head/hair and it is absolutely shocking how much is coming out! I will be bald in no time! It is shocking. My scalp is tingling. Wes says I look like a golden retriever who is shedding. I had to get a lint roller at the Dollar Store today when I was out with Victoria as there was so much hair on my back and shoulders. Oh brother! I think Wes liked collecting the massive hair ball from my hair. He put it in a ziplock bag. Yuck! I also let him cut a lock of my hair off the side so I can remember what my hair looked like. It is so sad to see it go. I never realized how much I love my hair. Typical, you seldom miss what you have until it's gone! As my hair fell out, I decided to let the kids cut & "style" my hair. They were keen! Victoria has always loved playing with my hair, so this was fun for them. I didn't mind. What did I have to lose?

The Dogs are Treating me Differently

Marley who is usually aloof and frequently does not have the time of day for me, is reassuringly by my side. Once Wayne gets out of bed in the morning, she has made a habit of coming up onto our bed & lying there with me. She NEVER did that before, even when I begged her to stay with me, she would not. As soon as I climbed in my bed, she would leave. Now both Marley & Ricky are my constant companions, which is sweet! I love my puppies! They don't care that I look ugly because my hair is almost gone.

Last week when Beth came over to help out, when I had my port installed and needed to rest, Marley laid on the floor at the entrance to our bedroom door and just stayed there. It was like she was my protector, guarding me. I was touched. The dogs certainly know I am sick.

What is Beauty?

Now that my hair is so sparse, and I am missing a breast and I just don't feel well most of the time, I wonder about a lot of things, but especially I worry about Wayne falling out of love with me because I am so rugged looking. He assures me he is good with the hair loss and I do believe him.

My friend Colleen wrote me this email to address the "beauty" question and I thought it was beautiful! She made me cry…. Sometimes you get the most understanding from people who you were not expecting! This is what she wrote on July 12:

Hi Sweetie;

I was just pondering what beauty means to me and this is what I think. Beauty is how you make your children feel when they are sad, angry, hurt or happy. Beauty is when you let your husband know you are proud of them even when they do something a little dumb. Beauty is the warm hug and kindness you show a friend and someone in your family. Beauty is when you help a stranger and do not expect anything for it.

When I think of some of the most sought after models and stars you know their beauty is only on the outside and that's just not enough.

So, although I can't really understand what it feels like to lose your hair because I have not been through it, I know you are one of the most BEAUTIFUL people I have ever known!!!!!
- Love Colleen XOXO

How do I feel about my mastectomy?

Of course first and foremost, I miss my breast. My breasts were one of the things on my body that I was proud of. They made me feel feminine, womanly, powerful, pretty and sexy. Being feminine is a huge part of my identity. My husband loved them too. I nursed both my babies with those breasts! I had fun flashing them more than a few times. They got me into trouble sometimes, but it was all in good fun! I have ghost sensations, now that one is gone, when I get a chill, or when something feels good, but there is no breast there to feel it, but my brain remembers. They were a great source of pleasure for me and sometimes I would venture to say, they were the "keys to the kingdom"! I will never get that back. All those wonderful sensations are gone forever. But I am alive! I am thinking of getting a proper prosthesis. I am mostly comfortable facing the world with my butchered & battered body – showing that I am battling breast cancer – if anyone looks. I find, unless I am showing cleavage, no one really seems to look. On the outside, most of the time I feel strong & a strange kind of proud for my battle, so I don't wear a fake boob. I feel like it sends a message that I am not less of a person with one breast. I didn't choose to fight this battle but I have been chosen so fight it I must. When I look into my daughter's eyes – I know I MUST fight. It's kind of a sad pride, nevertheless, if that makes sense. I am not looking for sympathy but I do look for understanding. I feel like I carry the message on my chest that – YES, it can happen to anyone! Even me! Even you!

On the inside, I do not feel good about my missing breast. I do feel embarrassed, defective, like less of a woman. I don't feel good enough for sex anymore. I don't feel worthy and I am so sad about this because I feel like I am letting Wayne down too, although every time I ask him, he says he is not there. Although I know he would like to have pleasure besides, DIYs... *(do it yourself)* I feel like my body has let me down. I feel fragile. I feel like even if we did get in the right headspace to have sex, that I'd likely tear up inside and have more problems. Something always hurts. Even when I try to get comfortable in bed, every position has degrees of discomfort. It's just a matter of how much discomfort I'm willing to deal with, and for how long.

I liked that breast, even though it was a little bit smaller than my left one. I'm glad the cancer is gone and it's good that it could be taken out, but without that breast, I do feel less attractive, less feminine, less strong. ...Less than my former self, for sure! I don't know if reconstruction will make me feel whole but I imagine it will make me feel better and I can pretend enough to convince myself that I will be back again. I often joke about getting up in the morning & heading out the door, with that feeling that I have forgotten something... Oh, my boob is missing! I wish it was not missing. I wish it was still there – but healthy!

9   Considering Reconstruction

My BC Sista, Joanne Stacey ~ Thoughts About Reconstruction:

After my mastectomy, the last thing on my mind was reconstruction!! Many would ask and assumed I would have it scheduled but I had no interest. The shock of a BC diagnosis and going through a mastectomy and looking ahead to months of chemotherapy, radiation and healing, I had no interest in thinking of anything else but HEALING, getting the CANCER OUT, and trying to get back to some normal?

My breasts were never a big issue and I was OK with the prosthesis and just feeling comfortable and looking well. I had been on vacation with a prosthetic bathing suit and I never felt uneasy with the fake boob? At times, it was hot or awkward but it was OK and no one could tell as the forms and bras are so much more comfortable and there is a nicer variety, etc. I was surprised the bathing suits were as attractive as they were too? I had many ask over my year of treatment if I would consider reconstruction but I wasn't too bothered and hadn't considered it? I met other women who had chosen reconstruction and as I became more educated and aware of what kinds of breast implants and surgery that is available, I took more of an interest but still wasn't sure I wanted more surgery and was more concerned for my follow up appointments and hearing my treatments were successful and I was cancer free.

It wasn't until my oncologist mentioned the possibility of reconstruction (18 months after mastectomy) now that I was doing better and had healed well and could perhaps think of considering reconstruction. Around this time, a friend of mine had mentioned her surgeon and how thrilled she was so I called his office and asked for a consultation to learn more.

It was one day a few months while waiting for a consultation that I looked in the mirror and thought I didn't want to look like this anymore as this is such a shocking reminder of what took place 18 months earlier! The scars were aggressive and I didn't like looking at this daily and feeling unbalanced and dependent on my prosthetic forever to look normal! I became more excited about my consultation and had researched more on the different surgical procedures and was confident that this was the right decision and time for me to do this. The more people I told, the more excited we all became and they reinforced the perfect timing and that my decision was good for me and they were so supportive and some were even jealous!?

I was never anxious before my surgery and asked my surgeon, Dr. Avram to give me as little of the many details as possible as I didn't need to know all about it. The less I knew, the better even though he was thorough and explained the procedure (DIEP flap and tummy tuck) and post surgical care and healing process. I was extremely confident and comfortable with him. Despite the intense week in hospital and a rough time of healing in the plastics ICU and a week at home, I regret nothing and would encourage others to consider this procedure. I have healed well and feel great about my new boob and the reconstruction I have had on the other breast in an attempt to have a chest that matches. I look forward to having the new nipple reconstructed soon too as I complete the surgery this summer ~ 2012.

Victoria asked a question – "Why cancer? Why me? Why us? Why anyone?"

This is such a valid question! Of course, there is no answer. But the question remains. It is a glaring statement of the unfairness of

116

it all. Why do we have to deal with cancer? Why don't we have a cure?! Why should anyone have to go through this? It just isn't fair! My children don't deserve this! My husband does not deserve this! We don't deserve this! My family does not deserve this! Why then? What am I supposed to learn from all this? Do I need more patience? Do I need to suffer more? What am I supposed to learn from this? That, I just want to know!

What about our sex life?? Loneliness ~ August 16, 2009

Can there be intimacy when there is "OUCHY"? I would be remiss if I didn't include how breast cancer has impacted our sex life. Sex is such an important part of our relationship!

To think I was concerned about an inverted nipple & now my entire breast is inverted and scary looking. It reminds me of a little old toothless lady's mouth, all pulled in through the middle, but ready to reach out & gum you – yikes! That must be such a turn off! Also, without that connectedness, for me at least, comes loneliness!

Sometimes I feel so agitated, alone and lonely. I feel distanced from Wayne. I miss our lives together the way they used to be. I want to talk more but I feel like he wants to talk less. Sometimes, I know he needs to get away so he golfs or travels or works later but that scares me too. Today when he got back from golfing, I was worn out. I did too much housework – just tidying up last night's and this morning's mess in the kitchen, the back yard, doing laundry & dishes & recycle runs, making our bed, emptying garbage, etc. I felt resentful that he was not here to help me. The kids were exhausting me. I just didn't want to walk out of the house leaving the mess, and yet I desperately wanted to get out for a walk. By the time I was finished what I wanted to do – just the basic stuff, Wayne got home around 1pm. (7-1) 6 hours! Yes, today I am resentful & I don't know why I feel this way! When was the last time I had 6 hours to play or have fun! Even a couple of hours would be nice! It seems he always makes time for himself to have fun (which I know is essential for him) but I am never included in that equation anymore. It hurts me!

I miss our Saturday night dates. At least then I knew we would give time, TLC and attention to each other. I just feel rejected. I don't know what is going on in his head but I know that the distance between us is affecting me. We don't touch as much. I wonder if because he knows that sex is not likely, he can't be bothered to touch me or show affection in a physical way.

I dragged myself through Staples to get school supplies for the kids. When I got home he had been catching up on sleep I think, so he hadn't left to get groceries yet. I walked in the door, flustered from refereeing the kids, and he walked out. I told him to please take a child, so I could sleep. I wanted to swim or go for a walk but I was done – exhausted. I slept until 6. He made a good dinner. He ate & finished first & immediately left the table to watch golf on TV. No conversation. Again, I felt hurt.

I struggled to clean up the dishes & the kitchen from dinner. What can I say? When I say I would like to talk, he says "What do you want to talk about?" Like suddenly I am on the spot, to come up with engaging topics... Then I come up with nothing much when I know there is so much we should be talking about. I don't like when I feel resentful because I love him & I don't want to hurt him and things just come out wrong & I don't have the resources to deal with the stress. I am grateful he made dinner. All I had today was a bowl of cheerios. I couldn't think of anything I felt like for lunch. Everything seems gross. All I wanted was a fruit smoothie, but I couldn't find one after the back to school shopping.

I don't like the direction we are going in. I don't know how to talk about it but I miss our intimacy. I miss our connection. I can't give him what would have been so easy to give him before. A simple b.j., or sex in its various combinations, used to be so easy. Now I hurt everywhere – never mind not feeling sexy... My mouth is sore from the chemo, and I'm afraid to think what would happen inside me if we did have sex. The dryness, "vaginal atrophy", as the experts call it, scares me. I don't want to feel carpet burns where one never wants to feel carpet burns! I never used to find reasons not to have sex. I don't like this. I wish I could get into his head & know what he is feeling. I just wish he would tell me and not be defensive. I wish he would communicate with me. Sometimes it's exhausting always being the one who tries to pull out the feelings and the information! I just feel so alone and lonely!

Relationships ~ It takes more than your breast! It takes a toll!

My sister in law Dianna, who is a breast cancer survivor told me that any issues a couple has, the hardships of dealing with breast cancer will take their toll. We have been dealing with this for over 5 months now and I am now seeing and feeling what she means. My issue is that I don't always assert myself in my relationship. I can be assertive and defend my needs in almost every other aspect of my life, but when it comes to my sweet hubby, I have a hard time. I don't want to be too demanding. I don't want to be a pain in the ass and I don't want to be one of those high maintenance women. I think this is because I have a deep dark fear that if I ask for what I need it will be too much for him and it will cramp his style and he will not love me anymore. However, it is eating away at me. It is affecting our relationship. I feel awkward asking for what I need and want. I have a very hard time asking him not to spend a day golfing when I need him and when our family needs him. I feel guilty. So I try to cope but sometimes, I need him so much it hurts. It hurts the kids who need him too. Yet, I know he has needs too and he has an essential need to play. This is his therapy, or at least I think it is. He is happier when he plays. I guess most people are happier when they have time for themselves with friends. Some days I feel bad and worn out from refereeing the kids and being on them to pick up their mess, etc. I need to get out too. I get cabin fever. Besides that, my needs for play are a lot less than his. It's just that I need him more than I want to need him. I need him more than I think he is prepared for. It scares me that I will need him too much. How can I tell him? I need to express my needs and somehow not make him think it is his fault – which is always how it seems to go...

What Distracts Me

I find if I focus on someone else or doing something for someone, it makes me feel better. With this in mind, I decided to plan a little party for my birthday but since I had chemo on my birthday, it would be for the people and their loved ones waiting for chemo and a thank you for the Juravinski staff. What I planned to do was serve cake to everyone in the chemo suite, along with pink lemonade, and pink peppermints. When I asked if I would be allowed to do this, they told me I could give cake to the staff but I wasn't allowed to give it to the patients and their friends and loved ones waiting in the chemo suite. I liked to picture myself cutting and serving birthday cake to the many people waiting for chemo, watching them smile, taking their minds off the inevitable for a moment or two.

Since I couldn't give cake to everyone, I focused only on the staff and I posted a notice in the chemo suite, on pink paper, with the following information:

There will be cake!
Friday, August 21st
Anytime after 8:30 am
In the Chemo Suite
Come before the cake runs out!

It's my 46th Birthday and thanks to you, I'm still here for it! Just wanted to say a big, heart felt Thank You to all of you Juravinski Angels! I'll be receiving my 5th chemo treatment, so please come & say hi, if you can! It will take my mind off the inevitable! Thanks! Hope you can find 5 minutes to stop by! Love & thanks! Carolyn Schreuer & family

September 7, 2009

Victoria's birthday today! She is 12! I can't believe it.

Feeling discouraged ~ September 25, 2009

It seems I have lost my ambition with this project. I don't feel so much like writing anymore. I feel alone & lonely & down. I feel weak. This is one of those days that I am just feeling that I am not coming from strength. I wish I was, but I 'm not.

So much has been happening to me, I feel I can never catch up. I feel overwhelmed by the thought of trying to capture it on paper. My eye sight is deteriorating and my brain feels foggy. Wayne won't be home until late & I need him. Stupid me again told him to have a good day & did my best to fake muster the strength to sound like I'm okay with the fact that he will not be home until 8 or 9 or whatever. He will not be here basically, for our Friday night. I feel like screaming, "What about me?!" I know my body is not a raving sex machine but surely he loves me more than that, but I am having my doubts, as I always do. I almost feel like I don't care about life. I wonder what I have to live for... depression is creeping inside me and I don't really care because I have hardly any spunk left. I need something to look forward to. I don't know what I have. I hate to feel sorry for myself but I can't help what I feel. I can't seem to stop crying. I feel like I have no control. I don't even have the motivation to go downstairs to the kitchen to get something to eat.

October 21, 2009
Life After Breast Cancer Conference

Dr. John Lamont
Chemo Fog

Wellwood Breast Cancer Peer Support Group

Testicular cancer?

Supportive?
Touch of kindness – necklace – symbol of health… Lisa
People say I'm their hero! Wow, who me?   I say, "You highly overestimate me!"

"I wish I could have hair like yours!"

Manicure & pedicure – Elizabeth, my red wig

Devil or Angel?
Halloween

Who's That Girl?

There is someone who looks back at me in the mirror. I hardly recognize her. She doesn't look feminine. She looks butchy. The hair that is sprouting on her head is full of dark brown bits and the blonde is barely visible. She does not have any eyebrows or eyelashes. There is a spot on her neck that sticks out from the port surgery and the line of the port scar shines in the light. This line is drawn diagonally above the purple bump that is the Power

Port. But at least below that there is a breast that I am happy to call my own. There is a strange landscape on the right side of the chest of this girl in the mirror. The skin is red on this side and very tender from 3 weeks of radiation, despite constant applications of Base Glaxal cream. It's a strange landscape and sadly, the breast that once happily rested there is long gone. I look in the mirror and the girl makes the effort most of the time, to smile back at me. I wonder where I went. Who is this girl? Where has her femininity gone? Will it come back? When? When will the hair be long again? What about the eyelashes? I see some more wrinkles and more weight through the middle. Can I get myself back? Who is this person? Do I really know her anymore? Who is that girl?

The Lesson

Kindness, patience, importance of noticing people, humour, priorities

What my Family has to say

"I'd give myself a B, or maybe a B-." Wayne

Thoughts on chemo, radiation
Fears, worries & Coping
Seeing me having my radiation treatments...
Counselling

Serenity and contentment when you least expect it

Comical moments
Hair – flipping my wig – A touch of Grace Day Spa
Getting charged less for a Brazillian waxing
Experiential learning
Affirmation whore

10 Emotional Support

Sharing Strength

One of the things that I have learned is that there is so much strength to be gained from sharing! I didn't realize how powerful this was before breast cancer, although I had an idea. Through my breast cancer support group at Wellwood, I discovered an online support community for Canadian women with breast cancer and the people I was able to connect with here, made a huge difference in my sanity!

I have always found it easier to write about how I feel than I do to just talk about it. When I write the words just tumble effortlessly onto the page. Writing has always been a wonderful therapeutic outlet for me, ever since I can remember. When I joined the "Sharing Strength" online community, I felt completely accepted, respected, listened to, cared about and comfortably secure. For me, posting questions, concerns, hopes, fears, experiences, supporting others, and sometimes just venting, became so easy. It was a safe way to let off steam and a real place to get feedback for every issue and concern that I had! Real women had already been through what I was facing and because of all the stages of where we were, we were able to help and encourage each other. Really, "sharingstrength.ca" turned out to be a wonderful, rich resource for me! Below is a post I wrote that I feel explains how much the strength I gained, meant to me!

I wanted to tell you that I read your posts and you have each touched my heart. Stevie and Bella and many of you "regulars" you continue to inspire me through my journey. Even if I don't always respond, be sure that your individual journeys have an impact on me daily. Frequently you amaze me with your strength and attitudes, you impress me with humour, kindness and sensitivity and you satisfy me with your open & frank comments about our BC journey(s)! Thank you for all that!!! This group has absolutely earned the aptly named title, "Sharing Strength"! For you "new" younger ladies, my heart goes out to you and I wanted to encourage you, if possible, to trust what is in your heart, and take it all one day at a time. It is all we can do. I was diagnosed last April (09) at 45 and I frequently am the youngest one around in various "Cancer" settings and here you are even younger, facing the battle, with young families and 30 something years of experience to cope. I really feel for you. It's never easy at any age, for sure! When I had my biopsy, a young female doctor took my hand (before the diagnosis was sent to the lab or anything) and she looked at me with very serious eyes and told me, "You will get through this." She was so caring & sincere and I often think back to that horrible day, April 6 - when I KNEW it was breast cancer. I can hear her voice and it still gives me hope.

I had a multifocal tumor, stage 3, invasive with lymph nodes involved and had a mastectomy in May, chemo from June to October, (8 treatments-"dose dense" every 2 weeks) and 5 weeks of radiation (25 treatments) in October & November. I am recovering and have just started an exercise & recovery program at the YMCA, which is great! I am hoping to begin the reconstruction process in March this year. My hair is growing back and my energy is gradually returning. There is hope! It seems like such a long time when you are in it, but looking back now, to all that I've been through, it feels like it was a short time. Crazy eh!

The hardest part for me, was the emotional stuff. I could deal with the physical stuff, but the emotions are what gave me the most pain. I have been seeing a counsellor who has helped me tremendously. I still talk to her every couple of weeks! Overall I would say, with that part of the journey behind me, that I feel empowered and I do feel enriched to have experienced it all. I am still coming to terms with what the experience has done for me, but it definitely made me realize that I am much stronger than I thought I was, and I am very grateful! I just want to ensure I don't miss any of the lessons, so I am constantly reflecting on what this has done for me.

On the positive side, going through BC gives you strength, empowers you and makes you realize what contentment really is. It's not always what you think! Of course, I couldn't feel this at the beginning of the journey, but I can now!

Keep in touch! We are all here for you! Take care & be kind to yourself!

As you can tell, in this post, I was encouraging a newly diagnosed woman. Just recently, March 2011, the website Sharing Strength is merging into a larger Cancer Sharing online community, called "CancerConnection".

What have I learned?
Life is precious – every life
Be forgiving – everyone is facing a battle of some sort
To be more patient
To drive more carefully
What chronic pain feels like
What it feels like to have your memory fail you
What menopause feels like
Dealing with pain
Trusting people
Always looking for the best in people
Taking time for the simple little things is so important – holding the door, taking time to spend with friends, waving thank you to other drivers,
Caring about myself and others is paramount

I'm stronger than I thought I was
Everyone has a battle of some sort & it's not a competition
Kindness is paramount - everywhere, always
What contentment is ~ real contentment…
The vulnerability of being dependent on others
Empowered to be able to face what ever I need to face
Deal with problems head on
How frustrating and aggravating boredom feels
Celebrate everything wonderful, at every opportunity
Appreciate those you love, tender moments, nature
Live! Bitter, sweet – feel it, live it, hold it, deal with it, let go
what you need to
Negative people have no place in my circle
Opened my heart even more to be sensitive to others
Not sure if I'm tough enough now to do my job, or maybe I will
be better at it now, I hope!
Ideas about why I am here… to write, to communicate, to boost
people up, to see the best in people

Feb. 15, 2010

I have a severe brain fog today. Not good. I hate that! The
difference is that I am feeling now that I don't really care
anymore about keeping my nipple. I just want it off and I want to
move forward. I guess that is the difference between my last
posting and now. I hope I am doing the right thing. Today I feel I
can barely think. I just want to run away from breast cancer and
leave it in the dust as quickly as possible. Man, this all takes so
much patience.

Today my eyes are burning. They were burning yesterday too. I
don't know why, unless it just has to do with wearing my contact
lenses. My eyes are tearing too. I am very unmotivated. I am
really having difficulty focusing on anything. Perhaps I just need

127

sleep. How am I ever going to feel up to working full time again and in my demanding job? At this point I just can't fathom it. I just can't seem to think at all. It scares me a lot!

My Reiki Experience (sounds like ray-key)
Feb. 17, 2010

I keep my mind open to whatever I experience and I want to take it all in, wherever it takes me. This was my 4th reiki session and I was feeling more comfortable with letting go of my worries and just soaking it up. Also, on this day in particular, I was feeling a lot of stress and pain.   Maria, the Reiki Practitioner, made me feel comfortable and as soon as I laid down on the table, pulled up the blanket, and the soft music began, I felt a wave of relief come over me! I had no idea what would transpire but I knew at least I would feel stress relief, relaxed and hopefully uplifted too, as in the last 3 sessions, I felt lighter, like a weight was lifted off my shoulders.

I closed my eyes and told my mind to calm and let go. At first it was racing frantically from thought to thought, as it usually does, and I tried to focus on looking at the insides of my eyelids. I let the music wash over me and the waves caress me. I could feel my head stirring feverishly at first. Then I felt the warm energy at my forehead where I imagine Maria's hands were. It was like someone stirred my thoughts with a silent electric mixer and the images began on the inside of my eyelids. First I was completely covered by blackness but quickly, the black began rushing around, mostly from left to right, and it changed to dark grey, swirling and whirling like storm clouds, the unidentifiable shapes rushed across the screen of my vision~ the movie screen of my mind.

Every time I tried to decipher what a shape was or what the colour was by looking directly at it, it would fade into my peripheral vision, just on the outside edges of my visual range.

Still the storm brewed straight ahead. For a long time, and what Maria told me afterward was about half an hour, the "show" continued on the inside of my eyelids. The black storm shapes which had turned to dark grey, and then lighter grey and the speed slowed down considerably. I felt my eyes tearing up and a tear or two escaped down the sides of my face and ran to my ear. I didn't move to wipe it off. I just let it be.

As the grey colours slowed, through the middle of my vision appeared several spots of bright indigo blue. It was as if someone touched their fingertips in paint and pressed colour into the middle of the page. It was the brightest, most unearthly and beautiful shade of blue, like violet or perhaps indigo with a light source powered behind it, as it broke through into my vision. It was calming and soothing and I felt stirred emotionally as the indigo took over from the dissipating grey. The indigo lasted for a little while, and it pushed the grey to the edges and off to the sides. Another surprise, after the indigo, came the most beautiful light colour of lime green, but more bright than lime. Again, it seemed as if this shade was created with a light shining behind the colour, as it shined through to me. It was healing and peaceful and I enjoyed the emotional journey both colours took me on.

Just as the green was disappearing, a sudden, surprising bright white or cream coloured light came up as if from my chest or my heart, up my throat, my face and to my internal movie screen. This was a forceful light, direct and powerful, full of purpose it seemed, although I don't know what its purpose was – yet. It was quick and strong as it washed up from my chest to the top of my head and it caught me by surprise. I don't understand this, but I will explain what happened just seconds after that wave of white light.

Suddenly I saw two narrow flames shoot up from what seemed to be my heart of my chest. The first one appeared to be about 4 inches tall and very white, mixed with a bit of peachy yellow at the base of it. Almost at the same time, another smaller flame shot up from exactly the same spot only it was about half the height and pure white. As quickly as the fames came, they vanished and the storm in my head was gone. It was a powerful emotional experience and one I don't want to forget. I can't explain it but I am seeking to find some explanations. After this, Maria continued with reiki on the rest of my body, but I felt, as did Maria, that my head needed the most healing.

She later said she was drawn to my head and usually, she doesn't stay with one part of the body for such a long time, unless she feels drawn to it, which in my case, she did. Maria said as she was performing reiki on me that she got an overwhelming sense of how much I am loved and supported! I felt so good about that! I know it's true.

After this session, I felt very emotional and in retelling my experience to Wayne, I couldn't help crying. It was a therapeutic kind of tears though and it helped. I think Wayne just thought I was nuts. All I can say is I know what I experienced and it was amazing!

Later that day, I looked up on the internet about colours in reiki and I read that Archangel Michael who serves on the First Ray which is the Blue ray and the Ray of Protection and Power. Archangel Raphael who serves on the Fifth Ray or Green Ray which is the Ray of Peace. I felt very humbled and honoured if this was the truth. I felt like I was touched by an angel. I am looking forward to the next time the Wellwood Resource Centre calls me to book another reiki session!

Two websites where I found information about reiki meaning and meaning of colours are below.:
www.usenature.com/article_reiki_colours.htm
www.treeoflifereiki.com/colours_of_angels.htm

Reiki is an ancient Japanese technique that works with universal energy.

"The Deeper Meaning of the Word Reiki
A different take on the word Reiki

By Bronwen and Frans Stiene of the International House of Reiki
One literal translation of Reiki is spiritual energy or universal energy. We suggest that Reiki may have another meaning - one that does not stem from a literal translation but rather from one's direct experience. When we practice the various elements that comprise the system of Reiki we utilize spiritual energy (Reiki). Practitioners are surprised when they discover in their practice that different stages exist within this spiritual energy. A path is unearthed and those who conscientiously practice the elements of the system of Reiki gradually see where it is heading. To tap into this spiritual energy, in it's completeness , is to have arrived at the advanced stages of our personal spiritual practice. To paraphrase the experience of receiving the full effect of Reiki actually means to achieve satori*. At this stage all our ordinary perceptions are transformed and we realize our true potential as human beings. Attaining this enlightened state of mind and becoming pure light is the ultimate goal of a Reiki practice. This is reflected by the mantra and kanji (symbol) that are practiced at the third and final level of the system. The mantra literally translated from the Japanese means 'great bright light'. So the goal is to become this great bright light by achieving a state of non-duality or satori.
*Satori means Enlightenment"

from www.reiki.net.au

11 Self-Esteem

My 7 Wigs & their Personas!

I have to say that despite all the physical hardships I endured, losing my hair was one of the hardest. Being a Leo, our manes are very important to us. Fellow Leos will totally understand! Being a woman, my hair was a huge part of my femininity! I felt naked and vulnerable with out, not to mention, cold! I did not feel confident, empowered or proud. I felt ashamed and ugly and self conscious. I felt like when people looked at me they felt shock and then pity. It made me feel like a poster child for a , "sick cancer person". I hated it. Wigs did help me to feel I could face the world and sometimes even feel pretty. It's fun and amusing to go incognito once in a while. Nobody ever recognized me when I wore Debbra, the long brunette or Cleo, the black bob. That was kind of fun!

My husband was brutally honest with me one night, after some "makeshift (cancer modified version) lovemaking, and he even told me that the bald head thing just wasn't doing it for him. He preferred I wear a wig. At least he was being honest. I get that, but if you have ever worn a wig, you will know that they are not the easiest things to wear! They are hot and itchy and they tickle your neck quite unlike your own hair does. Another thing I discovered in the heat of a moment, was that my wig, in order to be practical, needed a chin strap!

Picture yourself on the bed, trying to enjoy a few moments of love, and with each thrust you long beautiful wig slides further and further up your head in the front and further and further down your back, rising slowly and surely off your head! Not the look I was going for! Sometimes it's hard to think "happy" thoughts when your brain is saying persistently, "Scratch your head, damn it! It's itchy under this wig! Just scratch it already!" You try to ignore it, but eventually worries about where exactly your wig will end up, and the adjustments you need to keep attending to, to keep it reasonably on your head, manage to completely invade and sabotage any sweet fantasies, that were playing in your head when you were enjoying the moment!

A lot of people said things like, "Wow, must be nice for Wayne, going to bed with a different woman every night." I just laughed and encouraged this delightful fantasy, but the reality was completely different! Now you know the truth!

My Main Mane ~ Elizabeth
Practical yet fun, confident and daring. Stylish, No nonsense. Hip. Pretty.
Short, chin length, vibrant Red bob. I love red hair. Always have! Always will!
My grandmother had beautiful red hair that never turned grey, even before she died at 72. My best friend Susan has brilliant red hair. My Aunt Norma has beautiful red hair. I have always loved red hair so it doesn't come as a surprise that I am most attracted to this colour. Every time I wore this wig people everywhere would compliment me on "my hair". People always think it is definitely my own hair. I love that!

Godiva
Sexy, youthful, energetic, lusty, strong & powerful.
Long, layered strawberry blonde – more strawberry than blonde. Side part and falls down in loose gorgeous waves to my waist. Godiva makes me feel like I'm a Goddess. I love it! I feel like it begs to be worn with nothing at all except maybe a stylin' pair of white GO-GO style boots, perhaps a belt and a big confident smile! It's a lot of hair! It feels like a whole outfit. Maybe I should get a picture taken like that! Hmmmm.... This wig I ordered online from Wow Wigs in California!

Suzie/Hannah
Fun, sexy, daring, energetic, alluring and confident.
Long golden honey kind of blonde with bangs. I get noticed in this wig! It's a head turner. It's the blonde thing! People always notice blondes! The kids call her Hannah as in "Montana" but I always wanted to call her Suzie, after my alter ego, Suzie, the party girl. She gets into mischief and pushes the limits. Suzie loves to party and dance and has a wicked lewd sense of humour. She is energetic and funny and loves to have a great time! Leo's choice! Lisa Gyokery, who teaches in Hong Kong brought me 5 wigs in the summer and Suzie/Hannah, Cleo, Bonnie, Debbra & Roxy are the ones from Lisa! That was the most thoughtful thing to do!!

Cleo
Sophisticated. Elegant, sleek, confident, powerful, mysterious.
Black bob, shoulder length with bangs and it does remind me of Cleopatra. Posh Spice.
At first I was the least keen on this wig but since I've worn it a few times, I am surprised how much it shows my blue eyes! I like to think I blend in wearing this wig. People still give me lots of compliments on it. Although one guy actually asked me right away if it was a wig. Hmmm... not sure if I like that it doesn't look like me, but I love how it is so bold, and so different from my usual look.

Bonnie
Conservative & tidy. Cute. Practical. Wholesome.
Blonde bob, shoulder length, pretty, with bangs.
The cute Mom next door look. Bonnie Hunt. I feel like I blend in, with this wig and it really feels like me. It doesn't stand out as much, but it is lovely and a comfortable match.

Debbra
A touch Punky, a little goth potential, and blends in, initially.

Long brunette with bangs, layered like Suzie. Comfortable for when I want long hair, but I don't want to stand out too much. Incognito – no one recognizes me in this wig!

Roxy
Wild. Daring. Adventurous. Confident. Edgy. Bold. Sassy. Flamboyant! Attitude! Rule-breaker! Dominant. Deep seductive red bob with bangs.
Wilder shade of red than Elizabeth and more artificial looking than Elizabeth. Makes people ask if it's real. It yells colour, and so what, "I dare you!"

Dreams
Oh, the entertainment of the mind! I am a very visual person and I think this is why I see things so vividly, especially in my dreams. Also, since I have a psychology minor and have always enjoyed psychology very much, I like to do a little psycho-analyzing of my dreams. Whether there is any truth to what I conclude or imagine to be the meaning of my dreams, is irrelevant! It just provides me with entertainment and temporary feelings of sanity! I have always had vivid dreams and I can still remember some of my childhood dreams, especially "The Poison Butterfly" and many adventures flying around, but that is another story. In the past I have often been able to rely on my dreams to give me answers, insights and sometimes relief. If I have a tough day coming up, sometimes I will live that day beforehand in my dreams and everything that can go wrong, does go wrong. I learn how to deal with the problems. I face the worst case scenario. I wake up fearful and exhausted but it's worth it, because, as I live that "tough" day and everything goes perfectly! I gain the confidence to solve all that I am faced with, because of what I already experienced in my dream! Cool eh!

Homes
During the summer and fall, after my mastectomy, while going through chemo, I had recurring dreams of houses. There were 3

different houses but the message was the same. All three were large, beautiful homes that I felt perfectly comfortable in, and each home was my home. I would always be welcoming people in, asking them to stay, saying we had lots of room and suddenly in walking through my house, I would always be so shocked to notice that there was something fundamentally wrong with the structure. I always was taken aback by the magnitude of the problem and wondered how we functioned in this house, the way it was. I felt a huge sense of urgency and the thoughts were always the same, "Oh my God, we need to get this fixed! How can we live like this? How can we function in this house?!"

As I would walk through one house, I was always discovering the second floor with at least 5 (extra) bedrooms! All the beds were made and everything was left perfectly, as I had presumably taken care of it long before. Everything was tidy & organized, ready for company! Then I would walk further in the house and shockingly discover that an entire outside wall missing! I wondered how the house was able to stand with only 3 walls & a roof and my overall feelings were filled with the dismay about how we functioned with a missing wall and the urgent need to restore order, security and fix it all up!

The next house was huge too and there were lots of rooms and it always had a huge pile of laundry in the basement, and at times, the laundry pile was coming up the stairs. The basement was always dimly lit and that always annoyed me because I couldn't see well enough and I felt nervous about what I might be missing. I remember replacing light bulbs there but it was still too dark for my comfort level. Part of this basement was unfinished completely and behind a partial wall was all dirt and a completely unfinished or partly removed foundation! The upstairs of the house was beautiful and I felt comfortable everywhere but the basement and the missing part of the foundation and basement always unnerved me! I was always checking the doors and securing everything I could and when I came to the basement I was washed with despair, about not being able to live with this mess and the insecurity! Again, the feelings were, were filled with the dismay about how we functioned with a missing basement and foundation and the urgent need to secure my home and get it all fixed up, as soon as possible! It was overwhelming!!

The third house was a beautiful house too, although I don't recall seeing any of these houses from the outside. What was important to me in all three houses was all the inside and the feeling of comfort, the welcoming feeling and safety it provided. What stands out the most in my mind for this was the kitchen because the floors were all warped so much that it was practically at a 45% angle. Nothing worked right and it was a constant source of frustration. I would put things on the table and they would roll off, and yet I continued to set the table and place food on it for my family and things would just keep sliding and rolling off. Cupboards wanted to swing open and stay that way. It frustrated me greatly and I would think, over and over again, we need to get this fixed. The problem is that it was too big of a problem for me to fix alone. We needed to hire someone. How long could we go on like that, I wondered? How did it get this way?

This kind of structural damage, in all three houses, was very unsettling to me and yet I continued, determinedly, to try to function normally. I continued to cope although it caused me a great deal of stress and anxiety. I seemed to be the only one who was upset or frustrated by the difficulties of each house. If anyone else was, no one showed it or expressed it in any way. I remember thinking, how are we ever going to be able to fix this? How are we going to have the money? How will I convince Wayne that it needs to be fixed and we need to hire someone and right away!!!?? No one had my sense of despair or urgency. I seemed to be the only one who was concerned.

I had these house dreams over and over again! I realized that in each dream, the consistent thing was that I was the house! The house is my body, looks fine and tidy and to the naked eye, (upstairs) things are in place, but structurally, there is a serious deficit – my breast is gone! People are coming and going and everything looks like all is fine, but I know in reality, there is a deep, dark, nagging entity that has invaded the security and comfort and order of my home, that I (& only I) can deal with – the cancer. Oh sure, other people can help me and they do, but ultimately this is my beast to kill and my dragon to slay and I must do it alone. Despite the challenges, I am determined to keep functioning. I keep doing laundry, changing light bulbs, feeding my children, making beds, welcoming people into my home and I keep trying to function as normally as possible. It's all I can do. It's all I know how to do. I don't feel angry at all. I feel scared and frustrated and surprised and shocked! I feel a bit indignant too! How dare it?! But then I feel nervous and scared again ~ and tired, very tired. I feel tremendous kindness and love in the comfort of friends and family and their presence gives me great comfort and strength. They give me energy and hope and such great comfort! That is why I keep inviting them to stay. It helps me deal with (or perhaps deny for a while) what I know is there, lurking, waiting to cause me grief or harm.

Of course, this sounds just like what I was going through with the cancer. Part of my body was gone – my structure removed. I will never be the same. My foundation is forever changed and eventually I will get this fixed. Reconstruction is looming for me in April. I wonder what my dreams will tell me next.

My Body Fails Me

Most people, I think, have experienced this kind of dream. You are in a dangerous situation and you know it requires a "fight or flight" response. You go to scream and suddenly you have no sound or voice. You go to run or move and your body feels like you are in slow motion, unable to move as if you are trying to run in water or molasses! You need to rely on your body, and suddenly, unexpectedly, it fails you! These kinds of dreams have been part of my "entertainment system" for as long as I can remember but in the last few months, as I have been working at trying to regain my strength and stamina, beginning to do the "Canwell" (cancer rehab!) exercise program at the YMCA, they have been recurring. Perhaps it is a reminder that I still need to keep at it and do a lot of work to get my strength and stamina back.

I am walking somewhere, near railway tracks with my daughter and it is dark and windy. I am not wearing practical footwear. I am wearing high heels. Typical. Victoria is holding my hand as we walk against the wind and some unknown force that I feel is against the odds. She is depending on me to keep her safe, my little girl. Suddenly just on the other side of the railway tracks, a huge wall of black rises up several stories, like a steel sheet ready to wrap up and devour anything in its path. I see it first in the distance, as it envelops people, cars and buildings ahead of the direction we are walking. An adrenalin rush! I grab Victoria's hand tighter and we start to run. She can run but I can't! I look down to see why and expect to see that I am wearing a long tight skirt that hinders my legs from breaking into a stride. Yes, I see that skirt and I tear it up in the middle, front and back and expect without that restriction, I will be able to run. I still can't! The black wall rises up closer to us and I realize we will need to go to the right and get up on the hill, away from this thing, which threatens us like a tsunami. My brain kicks into gear amidst my panic and we attempt to run up the hill... I feel like I can only move in slow motion. I cannot scream so I try to communicate to Victoria with my grasp and my eyes. She tries to drag me faster. I feel like I am trying to run through jello. I am holding her back. I can barely move...my body fails me. I realize I can't depend on it! I am gripped with shock, regret and fear...I fear for our lives!

More Weird Dreams ~ But what do they mean?
Pulling it Out of my Mouth
(Cue the snake charming music! Da-na, na, na, na, Da-na, na, na, na, na, naaaaaa...)

As I am walking, I cough and feel my mouth and the insides of my cheeks stuffed with something dry and dense. Ick! I cough a bit up and it comes out like strings cut up and folded from a paper shredder. Only thing is it just keeps coming and some of the strings are metal-like substances. Like a never-ending ball of yarn, or a disgusting tapeworm, it just keeps coming! Ick!!! I want to be rid of it all! It keeps filling my mouth as it rises from deep within my insides. Scary, but I keep pulling it up and out of my mouth but there is so much. I cannot get rid of it all! It just keeps coming. I cough it up and every time I clear my throat, there is more. Relief, if it comes at all, is only temporary. All my energy is focused on trying to get rid of this horrible thing inside me! It's scary and overwhelming. I hate it!

Reflecting on this dream, I think this is how I visualized the cancer being blasted and evacuated from my body. I hated being the "host" for such a sneaky, slimey, disrespectful, disease.

Reconstruction – still thinking! March 4, 2010

If anyone had told me a year ago that I would seriously be considering getting rid of my presumably healthy breast, I would never have believed them! It's interesting and sometimes astonishing how things change with experience! I see both surgeons this month – Dr. Avram & Dr. Saunders. Both are booked for me on April 19 to cut off my left breast and put in place tissue expanders. They will work together on me at the same time. I think I would really prefer to get my left breast scooped out like a pumpkin, but I don't know if they can do that. Also, I want to make sure that I don't have a "party room" for breast cancer, should it decide to come back! The more breast tissue I get rid of the better my chances! I have a mammogram scheduled for April 7 for my left breast and I feel good that it will be only the second and yet the last mammogram of life. I want to outsmart the cancer! "Ha ha! You evil dragon! I have tossed away your house so you cannot live here anymore!"

I am 95% sure that I am doing the right thing by getting my left breast removed, but what will happen? Will I be able to keep my skin and my nipple? I'm sure the wonderful sensations that I used to thoroughly enjoy, will be gone forever. Also, it will be much easier to match up my breasts if they are both made of implants. I want to be proud of my girls again – someday! It will make me feel more feminine again. As my hair grows again, that will help too!

I said to Wayne the other day, "It's funny, I have often fantasized about receiving the attention of 2 men at the same time, touching me... having their undivided attention, however having Dr. Avram and Dr. Saunders operating on me at the same time, is not exactly how I envisioned it! Of course they are both absolutely gorgeous, but I will (hopefully!!!) be sleeping through all their "TLC:!

12 Saving My Sanity

I had to have a chapter on mental health because as anyone will tell you, facing cancer is as much of a mental battle as it is a physical one. I feel often that the mental and emotional aspects of facing cancer are much more difficult to deal with than the physical ones.

To physically have an important part of my body cut off, is a part of the challenge, but although I really miss my body being whole, I am grateful that the cancer was in a part of me that could be removed, without completely limiting my ability to function. Better a breast than my leg or arm or brain or lungs. I can still walk, dance, swim, read, write and have conversations, play with my dogs, write, and hug my children and love my husband.

Having grown up with parents who always told me to "keep my chin up" or "look on the bright side" and who saw depression and mental illness as not a disease or illness but a sign of weakness and a severe lack of will power, I had to learn to open my mind and develop respect for the wallop of a punch depression can have on a person, regardless of their strength of will power and determination! This has been a good lesson for me too. I have to credit numerous people and organizations for helping me through the difficult patches. I might have survived alone but I definitely wouldn't have done so well. Emotional support is essential!

If you're facing this, reach out to everyone and every source that offers you help! That's one thing I've learned! Not only does cancer test who you are, it also tests who others are! I discovered a tremendous community of love, support and kindness, far more than I ever imagined! Cancer brings out the best in people! I even discovered that a few people who I thought were at best, mediocre, toward me, turned out to feel exceptionally concerned and showed me incredible kindness and sensitivity. People came out of the woodwork to show kindness and support. Along the way, there were a few people who dropped off in their communication, and I don't take this personally.

I recognize that facing cancer is not a comfortable thing to do. Many people feel they do not know what to say and they don't know how they could possibly help, so they step back. Some feel overwhelmed and shy away. Some people are simply terrified and the only way they can deal with it is by detachment or denial. Some people worry it will bring them down or spoil a mood so they would rather avoid it and "enjoy" the mood! Some people who have already faced it in their families are incredibly understanding and supportive and intuitive and others can't cope with reliving that memory and cannot face it. I accept this and feel that life is too short to harbour any ill feelings toward anyone I love. Kindness and forgiveness are paramount. It's not someone's fault if they have difficulty dealing with cancer. It's very tough! Heck, you can't even buy a "Hallmark" card that says, "Sorry you have cancer. I don't know what to say or do. I feel helpless... But that really sucks!" What *is* a person supposed to do?!

Incidentally, I think "Cancer Cards" could be a niche in the market. I could design them, write them and Hallmark can sell them and give some of the proceeds to cancer research! It's one of my many ideas that I think is a good one but I just don't have the ambition and extra energy to market this.

For what it's worth, my advice would be to find it in yourself to reach out to the person with the cancer, and ask they how they are doing. Be prepared to listen. They don't expect you to fix things or have any solutions. Just listen! That helps so much! The most helpful things were things like, people bringing food, people offering to walk my dogs, people who would come over to sit and talk for a bit, friends and family who sat with me through my chemo treatments, people who drove me to appointments when I was just too exhausted, those who helped around the house, fixing this or that, odd jobs, sweeping the floor, weeding the gardens, people who made me laugh and people who came over so we could go for a walk and talk, and those who hugged me and held my hand, either physically or virtually.

What was not helpful were people who tried to make me (or possibly themselves) feel better by diminishing what I was going through or what I was facing:

Oh, you will be fine.
It's probably not cancer – you have no family history.
You're too young to have it anyway.
Oh, it's so good they caught it early enough, right!
Oh, hardly anyone gets a mastectomy anymore.
You look fine! When are you going back to work?
There's a 95% survival rate for breast cancer – so you have nothing to worry about.
Imagine the children that have to go through this!
It's not a big deal.
I know tons of people who have gone through this, and they are fine now.
It's not a tragedy or anything.
My girlfriend had a double mastectomy and her fake tits look great!
Who needs a breast anyway! It's useless!
Hey, you are soooo lucky, you get a free boob job!
OMG, are you getting a free tummy tuck too? That is worth about $8000! You lucky thing!
Fake boobs look better anyway and they won't sag.
Oh you are so lucky to be off work!
What do you mean you sleep-in all the time? Why?
Oh you must watch lots of TV.
How painful is it, really?
You look good bald.

Oh you must be soooo bored!
What do you do all day long?
What I would do if I were off work for that long is... train for a
triathlon, travel, climb Mount Everest, tame a few lions, fly to
Uranus, plant a rose garden on Mars ~ blah, blah, blah...

Ahhhh, ummm, did you forget that I am *sick and recovering from*
cancer?!

Who & what helped:

Obviously first & foremost are my hubby, family & friends &
neighbours who were supportive.
People who work at the Juravinski Cancer Centre ~ I can never
say enough good words about the care I received there!
Lynn Hyruink – CAREpath Oncology Nurse who called me every
Monday, all through diagnosis and treatment, and beyond!
Hurst Place – my amazing counsellor Kim
Juravinski – Linda Learn – Social Worker
Susan my friend who flew from Nova Scotia to be with me
through some treatment
Nurse Lisa – my friend & neighbour, who came to give me my
needles & hugs!
Lisa – my friend, & Nurse Practitioner
Sue – my cousin
Ann, Christina, Lisa & Kathryn in my peer support group
SharingStrength.ca – Colleen & the ladies on this online
community & support network
My School and the Sherwood community – my other family!
Many People who called me to check in and see how I was doing
VON Nurses who helped me, changed my dressings & talked to
me after my surgeries
Writing helped me tremendously!
Conferences – CBCN, Body, Mind, Spirit, October 2010
Reading helped me ~ it was great to escape into someone's story

13 Respecting & Accepting my Body

Although I have always had a battle with my internal clock that my body seems to prefer, I have given this desire consideration since being off. I always knew this but over the past few months, it is clear that my body likes to settle down to sleep well after midnight and it prefers to get up some time between 10am and noon. I don't like this but I have given up fighting it. Some things you just eventually accept. I wish I was a morning person and perhaps as I get older, it will happen. I think I would like that! Perhaps I was meant to be a bartender instead of a teacher!

I wish I could have been a hair stylist but I suck at styling hair. I wish I liked gardening, but so far I just don't! As for feeling feminine without a breast, it's really hard for me. I just feel incomplete. I feel boyish, masculine, butchy and I don't feel good about it at all! I can accept that my body let me down and I can accept that I have to deal with cancer. Now I am learning to respect my body more and listen to my needs. I take more breaks. I sit down more. I try to eat healthy, but sometimes I cave and eat chocolate and sweets. I drink a lot less alcohol, although I still enjoy it a lot! I think having breast cancer has taught me to realize that sometimes my body has limitations and I need to respect that. I'm not perfect but that is becoming more irrelevant. What is important is to love my body and be happy for what it does for me. Sure I want to look great and feel healthy, but I guess I will probably never be like those skinny 20 something women we see everywhere, and that is okay!

Always More Month than Money

The books and resources you read from the United States always includes a section of finances. Finances have always been challenging for me. Don't get me wrong. I seem to have exceptional talent for spending money. My hubby and I always joke, "Know your strengths!" Whenever I was reading, I always just scanned over this section because, living in Canada, I deemed it irrelevant. We have our OHIP health care coverage. I have my medical insurance through Great West Life at work. I will still get 60% of my salary when on LTD. I won't have to pay taxes on that 60%, I think. I will be fine. Right?!

Well as distressing as this is, I am getting used to my debit card being declined due to insufficient funds. I have even had my credit card declined now too. Yup! It's true! I'm not proud of this. Actually it's quite embarrassing, but I really suck at this and I am going to try to get better! So what do I do when I need groceries, gas, dog food, soap, laundry detergent or my kids need new running shoes, I use another credit card! It's bad, I know. Despite my overdraft protection of $3500, I more frequently than not, run out of money before I run out of month! I hate it! It makes me feel like crap! I feel like this should only happen to "bad, irresponsible, derelict people" and not people like me, but it does happen to me. It's worse since I've been dealing with breast cancer, as your priorities change and sometimes you feel you must get what you need when the opportunity is there – you have the energy and you are out, because you know that if you wait for a few days, when you might have the money in your bank account, you will not have the energy to go out and get what you need... It's like being prepared for a storm – you want to have supplies on hand instead of facing it being unprepared.

I avoid going to the bank. It takes a lot for me to get the nerve to face people there, because I feel they look down on me, but I suck! I get 60% of my salary once a month some where between the 18th and the 31st of any month. I never know exactly when now because insurance puts the money in whenever they get around to it, or at least that is my impression. I receive a letter each month, after the fact, saying that the money will be deposited some time between whatever end of the month dates and to call them if I don't see it… blah, blah, blah… As well, when you are on LTD, your health benefits are no longer paid for at all by your employer, so you can opt to pay for your insurance coverage yourself or choose to have nothing. I'm not complaining or anything, but to maintain what my family has become accustomed to for the past 20 years of my working life, it now costs me around $450 a month and that doesn't even include everything, but it includes a lot (75 per cent of dental care).

Finances – Only in Canada, eh!

Having breast cancer does take a toll on you & your family financially. Of course, we have the huge advantage of our Canadian health care system, thank goodness, but you will find that there are still, several financial hardships that you might be unprepared, for that accompany this journey. Just off hand, here are some expenses that really add up.

Wigs & hats - $300 – thousands each & up!
Prosthesis – aka: breast form – only one $400 (You can apply for the Ontario government to pay up to $195 toward it, after you've purchased it.)
Specialty bras – to hold the prosthesis $60-$100 each & up
Specialty swimwear to hold the prosthesis $75 & up
Parking at the hospital for treatments, appointments, etc. – about $10-$15 a day
Medication, not covered by insurance
One needle I had to take after each chemo, Neulasta, to help my body produce white blood cells, was around $2640, and thankfully, my health insurance covered this! (If my white blood cell count was not up to par before the next scheduled treatment, then I could have my treatments delayed or I could be hospitalized for a blood transfusion to help increase my white blood cells to enable my body to withstand the next treatment.)
Physiotherapy – minimum $50-$75 per visit, often 2-3 x a week –

needed especially after surgery to prevent "frozen shoulder" and help regain movement of arm and shoulder)
Creams and over the counter products to help healing from radiation – about $15-30 each
Traveling to other supportive appointments, meetings, services
Clothing to provide comfort and accommodate your physical changes; foods you can eat that make you feel better; extra vitamins; new glasses – chemo accelerated my vision deterioration

Heaven forbid you live out of town and you have to stay and incur even more expenses…yikes! It can be very challenging, financially!

I feel grateful for being established in my career with a good, secure job and family health benefits and long term disability insurance all nicely in place, ready to use, if and when needed. A lot of women I have met who have been diagnosed with breast cancer much earlier in life, such as in their 20's or 30"s, do not have this luxury. Many do not have secure permanent jobs with benefits. Many are forced back to live with parents. Many are left by their husbands because they can't cope with the stress that comes with taking care of your wife through cancer and beyond. Many have nothing secure to fall back on – not a job, or a house, or an established career or reputation. They are just starting out and are left extremely vulnerable because they need to stop their lives in their tracks to deal with and fight this disease! Many young women have young children to support and care for. Many young women have trouble getting hired after cancer because a prospective employer does not always want to take a chance on them – their energy, stamina and their health. No employer wants to hire someone who might not have the potential to produce as the next person, who hasn't had cancer. It's a constant uphill battle. I feel lucky to have been in a secure place, when my cancer started to chew up my life and spit it out! Many women do not have the luxury of such a safety net.

14 Choosing Reconstruction

Something to Look Forward To

What I have found in going through this is that having something to look forward to is essential. Picture the donkey following the carrot that is tied to the string at the end of the stick held out in front of his nose, to give him incentive to keep going. I need that, except I need to be able to reach that carrot every now and then!

For my mental health, I need something to look forward to! Never has this been so essential! Through the cancer journey, you truly need to have things to look forward to because some days it's difficult to keep going. You want to look at the stars but you feel your vision is clouded over. Sometimes you feel too sick and worn out to be able to lift your head up high enough to even look up. Those days, even the smallest things lift your spirits!

Receiving a card, especially if it has a personal note inside
Receiving flowers
Getting a phone call from someone who cares and listens well
Being able to get out for a walk, especially when you don't get rained on
New Brunswick trips & Derek's Christening
Florida Trip
Lunch with girlfriends
Dinner with Girlfriends
Afternoon Tea
Going to a movie
Date with my hubby
Shopping when I have the energy and some money
Every day past chemo is a good day
Every chance to celebrate (& eat cake!)

Philosophies I like:

I'd rather be having birthdays than not having them! - Lorraine Baatz
It's never too soon to be kind to someone because you never know how soon could be too late. - Mom
Change is always difficult.
Life is all about how you handle Plan B. - Angela Broadley
Life is not about waiting for the storms to pass. It's about learning how to dance in the rain.
Life is not a dress rehearsal. - Rob McDannold
If I can't do great things, I'll do small things in a great way. - Carol Spray, UNB Prof
It's more important to be kind than to be right.
It is not death, but life that tries us.
The wisdom is in the room.

What is the Metaphor for your life?

I've decided that this can be very revealing. You can ask yourself this question. You should. You might not like the answer, but at least if you ask, then you can realize where you are and decide to make changes. It beats going through life unaware why you feel crappy and resentful. It can spare you regret in the long run.

I have given this considerable thought and I have come up with a few that work for me. Mostly I am happy and positive. These are metaphors that come to my mind.

Sunshine – warm, comforting, uplifting, shedding light, illuminating, cheerful
A ray of sunshine separating the clouds – that optimistic view that others don't always see

A river – always in motion, energetic and full of life, a source of life and a means of connection to people and places, a source of entertainment and connectedness

A lion – strong, passionate, courageous, protective, nurturing, demanding, respected, admired

A soft, familiar comforter/blanket – needed, loved, coveted, held, warm, protective, comforting

A confession box – the one people come to tell their secrets and trust me to hold them in my heart, enabling a fresh start, permission to renew & move on

A soft, comfy armchair – comforting, secure, welcoming, nourishing, rejuvenating, peace and tranquil

A feast to nourish the soul & body – comfort, nourishment, pleasure, inspiring, fulfilling, desirable

A puppy – completely joyful about life, endlessly forgiving, energetic, loveable, contagiously enthusiastic, naïve, passionate, comforting, soft and sweet, inspiring, vulnerable, optimistic

A joy ride – entertaining, fun, full of life and adventure, good times, laughter, joyful, exuberance, thrilling, energetic, addictive, desired

A cheerleader – optimistic, energetic, fun loving, enthusiastic, supportive, loveable

A peacemaker – kind, caring, loving, comforting, benevolent, fair, supportive, intelligent, harmonious, valued, respected, admired

However, on a low emotional day, when I feel down, discouraged or depressed, other metaphors come to my mind. Sometimes I see myself as:

A piece of saran wrap – useful in helping others keep it together, but transparent, see through, strong for others but flimsy in itself, quickly looked upon as garbage, once used, easily & thoughtlessly tossed away

A autumn red maple leaf that has fallen off the tree to the ground – used to be glorious, colourful and beautiful, held in high regard, but now is rotting on the ground, stepped on and generally worthless, beaten down, ignored, left as dirt in the cold

Taxi driver & money dispenser – used by teenage children, demanded of, expected to solve all problems, jump when demanded upon, provide at all costs, fix everything, live to serve - and in all situations, immediately, as requested, disrespected, taken for granted

Referee, that no one respects or listens or hears or sees – making calls in vain, for nasty, unrelenting teams who do not value harmony, fairness and are just out for themselves.

Can opener – a useful tool for others, when they want sustenance, but tossed in a drawer and ignored when not needed, squeezed hard, full of expectations, unappreciated, taken for granted, and cursed when not in perfect working order and readily available

A sponge – cleaning up all messes, absorbing crap, keeping it all inside, squishy, full of tears when rung out, fix it & make it better duty

A hamster wheel – spinning at nauseaum, running & running to the point of exhaustion, and then still expected to run more, with the feeling you are getting nowhere

What my Son Wes, Had to Say

Wes was 13 when I was diagnosed. After we had the difficult conversation with the kids, and told them, I wasn't sure how they would react. It was tough news to swallow.

Wes later told me that at first he thought it meant I was going to die. He felt it couldn't be real. Then he figured one surgery

153

would take care of everything and I would be all better. He was surprised that it could be true, that I could have breast cancer, because I had always been so healthy. In his eyes, he had always thought I was so healthy, eating right, being vegetarian and exercising regularly. How could this be happening?

Ten minutes after we told the kids, Wes went online to research about the survival rates for cancer. He said I didn't seem sick. I didn't act like I was sick. I didn't look sick. So far, I looked the same. How could I have cancer? I think he was in shock and denial.

When he saw me in the hospital after my first surgery, the initial mastectomy, he felt awful and he told me he hated seeing me like that. I didn't seem like I was his Mom when I was sick. It really hit him hard. When I was going for my 3rd surgery, in less than 2 years, to have the tissue expanders removed and have autologous tissue reconstruction, "DIEP", Wes said that even if I was in the hospital for a week, he didn't want to come and see me. He couldn't bear to see me sick again.

What My Daughter Victoria, Had to Say:

I think my Mom's cancer brought everybody in our family closer. I think it made us stronger as a family. It made me feel stronger. We spent a lot more time together. I loved it when my Mom got Fruit baskets especially the "Incredible Edible" arrangements. The flowers were pretty. The best part was having my Mom home a lot more. She didn't have to go to meetings after school. I really liked that she was home. I liked going to the "Y" with my Mom. I liked going for walks with my Mom when she had to walk slowly, because of surgery or pain. Sometimes we held hands. The sun was always shining then.

The hardest part was seeing my Mom in pain. When I saw my Mom with tubes up her nose, when she was in the hospital, that was creepy. Sometimes it was hard to hug or cuddle with my Mom because I knew she was in pain and I didn't want to hurt her. I miss playing with my Mom's hair. I used to like to give her pony tails and braids, before it all fell out from the chemo.

It helped me become more aware about breast cancer. I never knew it was that common and now I see a lot more fundraising to do with breast cancer than I ever noticed before. I think I might grow my hair really long so I can donate it to make a wig for someone who has cancer. I want to help.

What Wayne had to say:

Wayne said that he honestly felt gripping fear, with the worry about how he could possibly cope with all this alone – the family, the kids, the house, life without a wife… He admitted that it was selfish but his first thoughts were for himself and how would he be able to cope without me. How would he be able to manage the day-to-day operation? Who could he get to help him?

April 16, 2010
Bub-Bye Boobie Party!

This is my last weekend with my left breast. I can't believe it! If someone had told me a year ago that within a year I would have both breasts removed, I would have never believed it! Now, here I am, looking fondly at my left boob, feeling like I owe it gratitude for what it has given me. It's kind of like how you look at euthanasia – when you have to put your dog down when he is suffering and is ready to die with dignity. It just occurred to me that perhaps we could have a bye-bye boobie party!

My friend Michele had a "Good bye Uterus" party with a cake decorate with a frosted uterus and everything. It was cool!

No one seems to care, other than I do. I guess it would be a party for one. My boob & me...

Chemo Brain

Forgetting words – the white thing that is wet and you put clothes in before drying them
Train of thought going off the tracks

Reconstruction ~ I Miss my Boobs!

Even though most of the time I can laugh it off, not having my boobs anymore, there are always a few sobering moments when I really miss them. It's the silly, playful moments when I have pangs of sadness sometimes.

When a chill descends over my shoulders and down my arms and I experience the feeling that my nipples are suddenly about to do their natural thing and get hard, a ghost sensation happens and I realize that will no longer happen to me, for the rest of my life. Reconstructed nipples will not react or feel the same. I don't think they will have any sensation, but hopefully, they will look pretty.

Sometimes, as my husband is cutting the grass on the side or the back of the house, in those little areas where there is privacy, I would flash him. Just my two boobs, hanging out, but he always seemed to get a kick out of it and I did too. I loved how, no matter what – even if I was in my pyjamas, he always appreciated the moment. Funny how the spontaneous flash of boobs can cheer a guy up!

Sometimes when I was saying good bye to him in the morning on his way off to work, he would be in the car, backing out of the garage and I would be hanging in the doorway, lingering for a few last glimpses of him before he left for the day. Sometimes I would flash him then too and as he was backing out, he would always give me a smile and a thumbs up and we would laugh. Silly... but now what is weird is the urge or thought to flash is still there. I have those moments when I think about this and my brain reminds me that there is nothing there to flash, except for a couple of large horizontal scars.

Something that would be scary for some people to see, but my chest now that breast cancer and I have duked it out! I do miss my breasts, but I am glad to be living, of course.

June 30, 2010

I just had my 3rd tissue expansion yesterday and wow, I am unprepared for this! The pain in my right side is excruciating. I can barely move! I've taken a valium to relax my muscles and 4 ibuprofen and a few hours ago, an oxycodone. This is the first time in my life I have taken valium! Still, the pain is winning.

I haven't even been able to sneeze because the pain over rides the sneeze. I've only had 1 sneeze since my surgery on April 19! The few other sneezes that my body wanted ,all got "over ruled" by the pain, and got snuffed out before their time.

I look at the clothes that need to go in the laundry, that we need to pack for our trip to New Brunswick. I cannot even bare to think about bending down to place anything in the washer or dryer. No amount of pain killers help alleviate this. I don't know how I am going to pack, let alone carry my luggage and walk on the plane. I am in complete agony. I don't know what to do!

July 1st, 2010 ~ Canada Day

I had to give in to the pain. I was waking up all night long, screaming whenever I moved the slightest little bit! It was brutal! Poor Wayne! Wayne called Dr. Avram and took me to the ER at the General Hospital. Fortunately, the associates of Dr. Avram were there and they saw me almost right away. Dr. ___ was very warm and understanding. I don't know why but I felt embarrassed for going there and having to have some fluid removed. It seems so trivial compared to what some people have to deal with.

Dr. A. made me feel very comfortable about it, which was very nice. She had a bit of a time getting the gigantic needle in place but eventually, after a bit of fiddling around and a lot of pressure on my chest, managed to get some fluid to extract. She took about 48 ml out of my right tissue expander and the relief was instantaneous. It made me realize that all that pain was just too much pressure on the radiated breast skin & tissue. Wow, who could have imagine it would be so debilitating?! Such a simple thing. It also made me realize that I cannot take much in my radiated side. It means I will have to go at the process much more slowly!

Bright Run

For the first time, September 2010, I decided to do the Hamilton Bright Run, to see if I could raise some funds for cancer research. (BRIGHT stands for Breast Cancer Research in Greater Hamilton Today) Since I did the Susan G. Komen run in Buffalo, New York, in June, I felt it was important to give something back to our community and the people who gave me such excellent care! I don't see myself as a runner but I was hopeful I could do the 5km walk. I was concerned that I might not be able to, but it was actually much easier than I thought it would be! I originally set my posted goal for fund raising, at $100 to match my goal for the

Susan Komen Run. It wasn't long and I realized that I was able to raise a lot more than $100! It was exciting! I felt like I was genuinely giving something back and that made me very happy!

Friendship & Sisterhood

The thing that impresses me the most is the wonderful, supportive feeling I get from being in the company of strong women, breast cancer survivors, and supportive others who care and understand! It can't be duplicated anywhere else but when these opportunities exist.

I had been working out at the YMCA since January 2010, so other than a break for my 2nd mastectomy surgery in April 2010, I figured I was up for the challenge. Wayne joined me, as our children had theatre and other commitments that morning.

Yeah! I walked 5km. and I was happy to have raised $1240 for breast cancer research!

My Boob Rocks! (not to be confused with My Boobs Rock! – at least not yet!)

Well it's mid October, 2010 now and I am still going through reconstruction. I was hoping to have my last fill on October 5, but since I have had to go much more slowly, it will take a lot longer. Some people can take up to 140ml per fill. Some take between 60 & 100 ml per fill. I have to be content with 45ml. The last procedure, the pressure started while I was still on the table and all I could take in my right side was 35ml, before the pain won. If this continues to decrease, I will not be able to pursue this method of expansion. I don't want to have to go with the DIEP procedure. I don't want another scar. I don't want the hip to hip scar across my abdomen that is part of this. I already have a c-section scar that I used to feel self conscious about. I feel cancer has left me with enough scars already! I have been robbed of enough and I don't want to give it anymore of me! It has taken more than enough.

How I Decided on the Reconstruction Procedure:

I did research on the TRAM flap, the DIEP flap and a little on others. At first I couldn't see how I could discard a healthy breast, but after the chemo, the radiation and all that I endured, I started to see my other breast differently. Although I knew I would miss the wonderful sensations that breast allowed me, I could no longer see it in a positive light. I now viewed my left breast as a potential party room for breast cancer. Once I saw it that way, I knew I would be ready to say good bye to it, too. I envisioned myself with 2 breasts that were similar in size, shape, and texture. Potential party rooms gone, I felt it might give me an advantage in fending off another sneak attack from breast cancer.

I also felt betrayed by my breasts. I had always loved them and they had served me well, nursing our babies, and giving me pleasure. Once I realized that one was harbouring a fugitive, my feelings changed and my trust was broken. When you pride yourself on knowing your own body, a cancer diagnosis sure comes as a shock, especially when it is so advanced and you had not idea such a party was happening, right under your own nose. It shakes your confidence in your ability to know your body and your faith in being able to detect anything that is out of place, or not right.

Why I feel Reconstruction is Necessary for Me

I know that for some women, reconstruction is not something they feel is necessary, or even desired. That is not me. I couldn't feel feminine without breasts. I never felt whole and I hated how my clothes looked on me. It shook my confidence and I felt butch. To think I wondered how I could be a "sex kitten" without long hair and now I had to find out how it feels to still, at times, desire to be that "sex kitten" without hair, or breasts and sporting several scars!

I heard a quote on "Criminal Minds" the other night. I liked it and I wanted to include it in this book. They said, "Scars may tell you where you've been, but they don't have to dictate where you will go." I really liked that!

I want to feel feminine, and I want back parts of my body, because it is possible. I often say to people who ask me why I would go through so much effort, time and pain, to have reconstruction. I use this analogy. If you lost your pinky finger in some unfortunate accident and then you found out that there was a surgical way that it could be replaced.

It could be reconstructed to look like your lost pinky finger and although it would never have the sensitivity of a real finger, you could end up with a realistic looking finger and you would look like you have 10 regular fingers again. Would you do it? Most people say yes they would. It's a very personal decision.

Expansion #9, October 20
(Not to be confused with Cloud #9 or Love Potion #9 – No way!)

This expansion was going to be bi-lateral (both sides) but ended up being only my right, (radiation damaged) side, as Dr. Avram was trying to "play catch-up"! I was looking significantly un-balanced with my left boob winning the race. The procedure was manageable with the usual degree of discomfort, but by noon – about an hour and a half after the procedure, the pain in my chest was starting to build. I didn't have any medication with me so I headed straight for the bottle of oxycocet I had previously opened on my bathroom counter. I knew it would be brutal trying to open it once the expansion was ripping through my tissues and super taught skin. Augh! It was brutal.

The pain left me screaming for about 30-40 minutes until finally the drugs kicked in and started to relieve me. I spent the rest of that day & night in bed, in a self induced oxycocet coma. Wednesday evening, since Wayne was working out west, the kids fended for themselves, my neighbour took my daughter to her dance class and picked her up and she also took my dogs for the afternoon and evening. Thursday another wonderful neighbour took my daughter to school, and I went directly back to bed. I took the medication, slept, drank a bit of water and tried to keep the pain from completely reducing me to a moaning heap of flesh, not even comforted in the fetal position. I didn't eat all day. I got up for about an hour to sit and check my Facebook and my email, hoping for a hint that I might be able to function, but then I was so tired and sore, I just returned to bed. I didn't even get in the shower until after 6 pm that night!

My "boob rocks" are a bizarre landscape and other than projecting small mounds of flesh from my chest, they look nothing like breasts. There are no nipples or areolas. There are two long horizontal pink lines across the middle when I have been cut. The flesh bulges out in whatever way it can and not necessarily in a round shape in the front. A little skin bulges to the side and where the scars sprawl across, the pink skin is indented and very tight. I look forward to a time unknown in the future when the strange, bizarre and battered landscape that is now my chest, will resemble even remotely attractive breasts.

They feel like boulders are strapped on my chest with a 10" wide and severely tight rubber band. The expanders dig into my ribcage, especially on my right side, when I try to reach down to shave my legs. The boob rocks are very hard and misshapen, like boulders I used to marvel at when I was a little girl. I always had a fascination with rocks! There is constant pressure and anything that requires the use of my pectoral & surrounding muscles is a challenge! Sometimes, opening a "child-proof" pill bottle is nearly impossible. Imagine trying to turn on a faucet or a turn a door handle or cut vegetables, or open a jar or even a water bottle. Imagine not being able to carry a full laundry bin or mop the floor, windex a mirror, or pick up your little 10 pound dog, lift a pot off the stove, wash a heavy pan in the sink...Even turning the steering wheel in the car and closing the car door are challenging and very painful. You do get used to the pain and after a while you anticipate it and you expect it. Every once in a while, long after a procedure, I have a painless experience when I perform a basic task and I am completely delighted! Last Saturday, before my most recent procedure, I was driving, running a few errands with my daughter and as I backed out a parking spot, and turned the wheel, I suddenly realized that I wasn't in pain! It was truly a wonderful moment! I almost cried I was so happy! What a brief moment of triumph to be pain free during a basic moment of life! Wow! I savoured it and now I think back on it, looking forward to another moment in the future when I might experience a pain free action again!

Reconstruction Frustration!
The expanders aren't working for me!

I decided to vent on the website "sharingstrength.ca". Thank goodness for this outlet!

Well, ladies, I'm here to vent! I hope you don't mind! I am feeling weepy today and I need an outlet. I'm not feeling angry yet, but perhaps it will still come. I don't know. I just feel like I got the wind knocked out of me and I just can hardly be bothered to pick myself up. Today I went shopping wearing my pj top that I had worn all night to bed, no make up, hair messed up, my teeth not brushed, not showered and I didn't care! This is totally NOT me, but I feel like I could care less. In April 2010 I had my second mastectomy (prophylactic), and had bilateral tissue expanders put in place. I have been going slowly with expansions as it has been very painful and I have been spending 2 days in a more or less drug induced sleep after each expansion to get past the pain.

Yesterday, I found out that my radiated breast side is at max and it cannot go any further. I still look like a size A and I used to be close to a C, before cancer. I was hoping that new breasts would be my only perk out of this deal. Now those hopes are dwindling too. Now I need to get the expanders taken out and I am heading for the DIEP surgery in the new year. It is a lot more surgery than I wanted, but I can't bear the prospect of living without my breasts. I am having twinges of regret for choosing to get rid of the "potential cancer party room" that was my left breast.

I feel like just slumping over and I am crying off and on all the time. (yesterday & today) I also feel guilty for feeling so upset about this, because not everyone understands what a big deal breasts are to me. I'm only 47. Maybe if I was 95, I wouldn't mind, but I do!!! It's so much more than vanity. I want to feel good about my body. I want to feel girly and feminine again - if that is ever possible. I don't know why I'm so upset, but I just am. I feel like I'm falling apart.

I've done so well through all of this and now this crap is really bringing me down. I invested 8 months of time, effort and pain into this and now, I will still end up with God knows what, a body full of scars & cuts, savagely desecrated by cancer. I know I should feel grateful that I'm still alive, and that I have a wonderful family, but I feel so incapicitated by this set back. I'm so sick and tired of all this. When am I ever going to feel good again? I wonder if I should book an appointment to see a counsellor... well, I can't be bothered... sorry this is so bleak, and not at all encouraging, but I need a safe outlet for these thoughts that no one really understands, unless they've been there.

15 Finding Another Lump

Finding another lump ~ December 2, 2010
What my (arrogant and idiotic) oncologist had to say about it:

"Stop *looking* for trouble!"
"You need to develop an attitude of healthy *denial*!"

I always say that my Oncologist did his job when he saved my life, and credit him with that. However, perhaps I expect too much from him, when I think he should care about me as a whole person, not just a breast cancer case. When I went to see him recently to have a small lump checked out - 17 months after my initial diagnosis, he was clearly upset with me for getting reconstructive surgery. (I had told him last time I saw him, that I was going to get reconstruction as soon as possible, so it's not like he was surprised.)

He told me in a condescending way, to "Stop looking for trouble." and that I needed to adopt an attitude of "healthy denial". He would not call my tissue expanders anything except "those things". He asked why I bothered to see him and why didn't I see my surgeon instead. He said he couldn't do anything for me. I asked him if I could be referred for an ultrasound to check out the lump, and he said no. He insisted that he could not feel my tiny lump in the same area as my original tumor. He told me he couldn't do anything for me anyway, because of the tissue expanders.

He said even if the cancer had returned, all he could do was "buy me time" and try to give me some quality of life.

I wasn't devastated, because I can handle it, but I wasn't impressed with his uncaring, condescending attitude toward me. I apologized for coming to see him and "being a pain", but I told him I wanted to be proactive and get "it" before "it" gets me again! He said if there was a problem/cancer, that I could wait a few more weeks and it would make itself known. Otherwise, leave it alone... I felt like I had completely wasted his time and mine. I felt dismissed, childish, stupid, disrespected and a little angry.

I asked my Plastic Surgeon to be referred to a new oncologist, as I see no point in continuing with an oncologist who clearly does not care about me as a whole person and who has no respect for my decisions and hopes/dreams to feel good about myself again. I'm only 47 and I feel like I want to live my life now. I don't want to wait around for reconstruction just in case cancer decides to return. What is the point of that?! What do you think? Do you have any suggestions for me? Everyone else has been great but this recent experience has left me with a very bad feeling.
16 Jan 2011

January 27, 2011

I met with my counsellor, Kim today. I was feeling frantic and mentally scattered and fragile regarding the surgery. Wayne being away doesn't help me because I have no one to talk to. Kim always helps me feel better and sane and she helps be stay assertive and proactive, while listening to myself and respecting myself! She said it's normal and expected to feel scattered and scared before surgery. Who knew?! Well, now I know!

If I could provide a wish list from my perspective, as a person going through cancer, the following things would be helpful:

Just listen to me & ask me how I feel ~ really. Don't try to fix, or correct or suggest that you know how I feel. You don't, but that's okay. I don't expect you to.

Don't dismiss my feelings and tell me that I need to be positive. I know that already. I need to accept my feelings and I need you to accept them too.

Don't tell me about your Uncle Fred who had prostrate cancer and just did blah, and is fine now. This is totally different! Even every breast cancer is different. There are so many variations.

Don't try to diminish my worries and fears by telling me a blanket statement like, "I know you will be fine." Listen.

Sit with me.
Make us a cup of tea, or a nice cold drink and put it in a fancy cup or glass, even if it's just water.
Do something constructive like:
Take my kids out for a while to do something fun.
Take pictures of the activities.
Take my dogs for a walk.
Brush the dogs.
Toss a load of laundry in the washer or dryer, or fold it.
Make dinner for us.
Drive my kids to an activity, or pick them up.
Read to me – something of interest in the paper, or anything.
Rub my back, or shoulders, etc.
Say something real and sincere.
Let me borrow a good book.
Brush and/or style my hair.
Get a few groceries for me.
Cut up veges or fruit so it's ready & convenient to eat.
Unload or run the dishwasher.
Clean a bathroom.
Take me out to see a movie.

Take me out for dessert.
Go for Afternoon Tea in a cute Tea Room, like "Taylor's Tea"
Room in Dundas
Go for a walk with me.
Change a bed.
Wash the floor.
Vacuum.
Clean or dust anything.
Water the plants.
Fix something that needs repair.
Go with me for a Pedicure and/or manicure.
Paint my nails.
Go to a yoga class with me.
Play some great, upbeat music.
Dance crazy with me, if I can do it, or if you can!
Cover me in a blanket if I'm cold.
Sit with me while we look out over the Hamilton Escarpment and
simply enjoy the view!
Go swimming with me or just float around in the pool with me!
Drive me somewhere – especially anywhere where I can see the
water & even better if I can see sail boats.

Another thing on this "journey", I found myself contemplating, as
most women on this path seem to do, what is my purpose in life.
I even bought the book *The Purposeful Life* and I tried dutifully
to read the meditations and suggestions.

I wrote my list of what I believe to be my purpose in life at this
time. If you haven't considered your purpose in life, I hope you
don't have to be duked out by breast cancer to consider
something so important. Someone said a purposeful life is a life
with purpose, but I want more specifics! What came to my mind
initially was:
To comfort,
To show kindness

To write
To feel & empathize
To listen
To care
To help others
To make a difference (inspired first by my friend & dental Hygienist, Jasmine)
To encourage
To be patient
To be understanding
To stand up
To set an example, in a gentle way, not a pompass way
To protect
To seek justice, especially for those who need help standing up for themselves

I don't consider this a complete list but it's a good start.

Reconstruction
There's a lot to say about reconstruction. Physically, emotionally and otherwise...
I had the DIEP surgery on Feb. 28, 2011. It was a 9-hour surgery with 3-4 hours of recovery and I spent Monday to Saturday in the hospital. (DIEP - deep inferior epigastric perforator flap) using your body's own tissue to reconstruct your breasts, also known as autologous tissue reconstruction — reported to be the most complex reconstructive option. As I say, not for the faint of heart!

In a nutshell, I can tell you that in a way, it sounds like a dream! Years ago, I used to joke about the bit of weight that found its way to my mid section, especially after the birth of our children. I used to say, "If only I could take the weight from down here, *(my hips, belly, etc.)* and just move it up here!" *(to my breasts)* "Oh, wouldn't that be just great! Wouldn't that be amazing! Can you imagine of I could do that?!" Blah, Blah, Blah...Ha! Ha! Ha!

Silly me again! I get to eat my words! That is basically what this procedure does. Most will say you get a "bonus tummy tuck" and they make new breasts out of your own skin, flesh and fat from your abdomen, specifically the area below your belly button and about your pubic bone, hip to hip! Sounds easy, right! A dream come true, right?! Miraculous it is, but easy, it is NOT! I got to do just that and boy I was in for a lot more than I realized. I may be wise in a lot of ways but I have decided that I am definitely stupid and naive when it comes to being a patient and recovering from surgery. Boy, what a dummy! I really need to be more careful about what I wish for!

This is the email I sent out to my family and friends after I got home from the hospital.
Oh, it's great to be home! I just wanted you to know that I got home from the hospital yesterday afternoon, Saturday, March 5, 2011, and am doing pretty well, especially considering what I have been through and how far I have come, even in the past week. I hope this is not TMI (too much information) for you. I apologize if it is. You can feel free to skip any parts that are too gross. Hardly anything seems gross to me now, so gauge on reality is skewed. However, if you find yourself on the edge of your seat, craving more gory details, (ha! ha! - not likely) please feel free to ask me anything specific, and I will get back to you!

I had all 4 drains removed before I left the hospital, so that was a huge relief, even though the nurse who removed them had never actually removed a drain before in her life. I realized this after she removed the first one an then I gently coached her through the last 3! Fun! Thanks to Lisa, who encouraged me to "pick up my stretcher and walk" (with the aid of a walker!) on my swollen marshmallow puffed legs and feet, for the first time, late Thursday afternoon! I was on oxygen until Thursday morning, as it was very intense for a while. I was reacting to the morphine and "was very far away". I am feeling pretty good, staying on the pain med drugs regularly. Believe it or not, this is the abridged version of the story, but Oh, there's always a story, isn't there! Had my first BM in a week today, so that was a huge relief. (Definitely TMI? I warned you!) I wear a wrap around my middle and only take it off for showering. I call it the squisher. I'm quite sure it was invented by a man. It's absolutely horrible! No woman would invent such a torture device! I'm not sure how long I have to wear it for - perhaps 2 weeks or longer.

Apparently the surgery went very well. Nine hours in the OR & 4 hours in recovery. Seems that out of the *(estimated)* 189 people in the hospital who came to take a look at me, and my "new girls", about 187 said they look great!!! To me, even though they are all cut up, I am happy just to have a part of me back in place. I think I am close to my previous size, so that makes me happy too.

Of all the things I said I wanted from this hospital adventure, the ONE thing I really wanted was a private room and we were happy to pay the extra $30 a day to top up to that, as we have semi private coverage through my health insurance. Of course, there were no rooms available, so I ended up in the Burn Unit of the Hamilton General, a ward room with 3 men, and what started out as a nightmare, worked out well in the end. It's not that I don't love men, it's just that this trip was all about my lady bits so I really didn't think they would want to experience what I had to deal with.

I entered the room from "recovery" by first having the porter and a nurse crash the head of my bed against the door frame and immediately was brain assaulted to the blaring awful sound of television - some fighting, sportish, hurting people, screaming type of show! I immediately started crying "NO, NO, NO, NO, I can't go here. Please just take me to the morgue. Please take me out to Barton Street. Please anywhere but here... I can't stay here. I can't deal with this!" etc. (not pretty-at the peak of weakness and vulnerability!) I was crying and felt completely wrecked and defeated. I was so stressed! It was a horrible experience and after having roomed with 3 guys after my first mastectomy, I did not want to repeat those fears and horrors. After the oldest guy (Lesley- who actually turned out to be a great guy) learned to use his headphones for his blaring TV, the following night, I managed. It's a good thing my parents trained me early in life to sleep when you are tired, regardless of any noise or loud, construction volume type snoring!! One guy was allowed to escape at some point and it turned out okay for the 3 of us after all. Bill, Lesley and I had some good conversations when we were awake and Bill and I spent quite a few snickers over the hilarious sounds Lesley created as he snored about 21 hours a day, and the other 3 hours he kept begging for sleeping pills, but they would not give him any! The guys were good, despite their suffering from burns.

I was very closely monitored for the first 48 hours (72 hours?) and Wednesday *(Well, not sure which night it was really - 1 night or 2 nights post op - Hmmm... who knows for sure!)* when I sunk low as I was only measuring about 47 per cent oxygen in my blood, when it should be about 98 per cent. My nurse Lori told me afterward that she would give me my medicine to take and I would fall "asleep" before I got it to my mouth. I was on IV and getting pain meds, fluids and antibiotics on that, and we were topping up pain meds orally too. I was barely holding on. All I can tell you for sure is that I felt super lethargic and very far away. I felt so far away, I wasn't even sure I would be coming back. Every time I did wake up in that hospital bed, it was not from lack of wishing I was anywhere but there! Luckily the light I saw was on the hospital room ceiling, not the "Pearly Gates". Ha! Ha! I was "dreaming" I was meeting Vesna for a "frapaccino" (which I don't even drink) in a cute little bistro place and just as we were about to sit down, someone called me back and I was back in the hospital bed, getting blood pressure measured, vitals taken, and getting poked with needles. Ugh. (I wonder if those were my personal "Pearly Gates"?!)

It was incredibly tough and I never want to have to go through anything like this again. My boobs look okay to me and are so much more comfortable, now that the rocks have been removed. Phew! At this point, I'm not sure if I will go for any more of the steps in the reconstruction process. Hard to say.

For now, I honestly feel like I'm at my limit of what I can take. I did get a blood clot in my legs, a one time appearance from a Dr. Bradley informed me, and they were worried I would stroke out, but they treated me in time. Had a CT scan afterward, legs ultrasound, chest x ray, and luckily my chest was clear from blood clots. Now, I can't walk and can barely stand for a short period of time. I'm just hobbling around, but keeping up with the pain meds helps.

My body is leaking and itching, and I'm moaning and groaning. I'm still very swollen. I've had lots of allergic reactions, mostly major skin irritation to hospital tape, etc. What added a lot to the discomfort is the fact that I went into the operation with a bronchial cough, which still persists. If you have ever had abdominal surgery and needed to cough afterward, you know how painful that is. I am sleeping in a chair because I can't lie down, but hopefully soon I will be able to find a comfortable position in bed. Wayne, Victoria & Wes are helping me tremendously and I am very grateful and blessed to have my family, friends and neighbours who do so much for us! I'm nursing all my wounds, and getting a wee bit stronger every day.

Thank you to my sweethearts who have come to see me already! Don't worry about getting in touch. Call me anytime! I would love to hear from you. If I'm asleep, someone will tell you, and I will do my best to catch up with you a bit later. Thank you so much for all your care, concern, thoughts, kindness and prayers. I hope this email makes sense. If it doesn't, I will blame the pain meds. Take care & thanks for everything.

Two weeks past surgery, on Sunday, March 13, I experienced a peak of despair, mentally and physically. This is what I wrote to my counsellor.

It will be 2 weeks tomorrow since I've had the DIEP breast reconstruction operation and although I am feeling better, I still feel like absolute crap!

I had some difficulties in the hospital with my oxygen dropping to 47 per cent post surgery and I think the morphine pain pump was a curse. I had such a bad reaction from it! I am still itching all over. My body is covered with scratches and tiny scabs, with me being driven insane, feeling the absolute necessity to itch...
Also, I am still swollen - ankles, legs, abdomen, etc. from all the IV fluid, & drugs I received. Ick! I feel like someone pumped up my belly with an over filled basketball. Pants which were considerably too big for me before surgery, I cannot get to within 6 inches of closing across my belly. Yikes! Could I be the first woman to have a "tummy tuck" to make my new breasts, and end up with a much larger stomach?! I sure hope not! I am covered in raw skin that is the result of friction blisters from the abdominal "squisher" thing (like a velcro & fabric girdle) that they put on me the day of my surgery and I wore 24-7 (except for a couple of showers) for 8 days until I just couldn't stand it any longer. I am blistered at the tops of my thighs and the top on my chest, under my new breasts.

I'm still bleeding periodically around the stitching around my breasts and leaking a bit of fluid, as all my drains were pulled out in the hospital. (by a young nurse who had never removed drains before, so I had to coach her on the last 3! Yeesch!)

What bothers me now is the feeling that I am pulled together through the middle, which I am, of course, but it prevents me from standing up straight. I can sit but standing & walking or lying down, I need my knees bent. So I walk like a 90-year-old person, hunched over, with all the pressure on my lower back. Ugh! Of course, that adds a lot of strain to my neck as well. I can only sleep on my back so I am also desperate to feel comfortable in my bed, but that feeling, if it comes, is very temporary. As well, my cough that persists from bronchitis I developed the week before surgery makes my abdomen feel like it is going to rupture and explode. Some times when I cough, I expect to see the free flap breasts, flying across the room, from the pressure that builds up inside me. For my cough, it would be good if I could sleep on my side but because of the surgery and the stitches hip to hip, it hurts way too much to endure!

I don't want to complain but I desperately want someone to tell me it is all worth my while! The expanders were not working for me, as you know, and I hated their hardness and as well, they did not expand sufficiently for me because of my radiation damaged skin.

My radiated side even ruptured the weekend before my surgery, likely because I developed a harsh bronchial cough, and I leaked out a hole that tore open in my radiated skin, as well as inside my breast and all around it. It was incredibly painful! So I'm glad to be rid of those tissue expanders.

I am going stir crazy, hoping and trying to feel better. I just want to be able to at least go for a walk, but I was exhausted just going to our mail box today and it is on the side of our house! I was pretty fit before the surgery and my cardio was good! I am scared and shocked at how much I have declined in the past 2 weeks! Do you think I am being hard on myself or perhaps I am experiencing a tougher recovery - who knows why.

I can't sleep through the night either because I wake up soaking wet with sweat, itchy, and uncomfortable having been in the same position on my back for 4 or more hours, and I have to strain to get out of bed to pee.

I can't drive. Otherwise I would come and see you. You always make me feel like I'm okay and not insane! Today I really feel depressed and like I am totally losing my mind! Nothing I love is fun anymore. I look forward to nothing! I can't do hardly anything. Nothing appeals to me. I don't care about anything. Even typing on the computer hurts my back a lot! I feel like I'm going insane!! I feel trapped. I begged Wayne to kill me this afternoon. I was joking but the prospect did have some appeal. Of course he wouldn't because he doesn't want me to leave him with this mess! :) I just cried and groaned and tried to move from chair to chair. I feel so incredibly discouraged and if I don't see/feel sunshine soon, I am quite sure I will shrivel up and die.

I hope this wasn't a decision I will live to regret. I thought I couldn't feel happy in my cancer battered body, but I seem to be in worse shape now, even though the plastic surgeon says everything looks "excellent"! Yikes! I'd hate to try to imagine looking "bad"!

If you can get a minute to call me or drop me a line, I would be very grateful. Sorry to be so needy and such a whiner. I feel guilty even complaining about my woes when those poor people in Japan are fighting for their lives. Man oh man, that kills me!!! So sad, it rips my heart out! How do they get past that - ever?!

Advocacy

I used to think that advocacy was not for me. I just want to live my life. I just want to get my life back – my pre cancer life! Yes, that's it! That is what I want. Now that I am coming up to 2 years since my diagnosis, April 6, 2011, I realize that nothing is further from the truth. I realize that getting to this point past cancer is not about being able to close a door and run as far away from it as possible. I realize that a switch is not going to turn off and my life will resume, happy and healthy as I thought it was before cancer.

My perception has changed. Cancer will always be a part of me now. It is not something I can run away from. I can't lever it behind in the dust. I can't bury it in the ground and emerge without it. Cancer has made me who I am today and I am actually proud of the woman I am now. It will always be a part of me and that is forever. Even though it was tough, I don't want to forget about it. I don't want to dwell on it but being able to embrace and accept this experience will allow me to do things and feel thing and help others like I would never have been able to do, if not for this experience. Like I always say, experience is the best teacher!

My cancer experience enables me to empathize with others and support them in ways I would otherwise not know how. It has filtered into every ounce of my being and I am forever transformed. It has left me with an intense desire to "give back". I always had the desire to give but now the difference is I have the "tools and the experience". I feel equipped and empowered to help others.

When I was going through treatments, I thought about advocacy as something on someone's political platform, a token, or something someone might pay lip service to but never really carry it any further. I knew I could never invest my time or energy in something like that. That was my understanding of advocacy. I also knew then, after I took care of what I needed to do, and gave something to my family, there was nothing left to give.

Now I am experiencing advocacy in a whole new light. I wish I had attended one of the advocacy work shops at the "Body Mind Spirit" Conference, but even then I didn't feel I had it in me to give that much. Now, it seems that I am falling into advocacy opportunities and I am loving it!

Sharing Strength

OMG, OMG! I had no idea Sharing Strength is closing up shop! I feel stabbed and a tad frantic! What happened?! Who will I vent to? Who will I talk to? Will we still have somewhere to connect? This site has helped me so much in my BC path! What will I do now? I truly feel at a loss! I didn't get an email until tonight and it upsets me a lot! Will the archived messages be accessible? I often sign on to read the wisdom from other women! It helps so much! I feel like one of my important resources and supports has been snuffed out!

Of course, thank you to all you lovely ladies who helped and encouraged me and gave me advice and support! It means everything to me! All the best to each of you in your journeys and lives! Take care & God bless each and every one of you!

Sorry, I really don't know where to post a message like this, but Colleen, I hope you see this too! I feel so sad - like I just lost a good friend.
Take care all you beautiful women!

Here's to survivorship and advocacy for breast cancer everywhere! Be strong ladies!

Love you & thanks again for everything you have added to my life!

Lots of love Suzie & aka: Carolyn
Posted by Suzie on 20 Mar 2011 9:19 PM

Post DIEP Surgery

Today is nine weeks past my DIEP surgery and I am coming along well, I think! I feel a lot better and some of my energy is returning, as long as I get enough sleep! I am now able to walk a couple of kilometers and feel good! The first 2 weeks was absolute hell! I don't even know how I got through that, but if I had the choice, I would have asked to be in an induced coma to get over the worst of it! Ugh! It was even more horrible than I could have possibly imagined!

I felt trapped in my body – a slave to my inability and lack of mobility. It's humbling and humiliating to be unable to take care of yourself and to have to depend on others for your basic needs. Going through that, has given me more appreciation for what older people have to endure and what injured people have to overcome.

On the positive side, the bumps now on my chest that used to be my belly, are starting to feel like breasts to me. I love that they are my own flesh and skin and they feel more natural. Those tissue expanders that were like rocks strapped to my chest, are gone and I am very happy about that! My incisions are healing and there are no open areas now. I still have a difficult time moving from horizontal to vertical and sometimes need a but of help. The 20 inch incision I have from hip to hip, is healing well now too but internally, I still feel tenderness and discomfort, especially at the end of a day where I have been active…

Editor's closing note: Unfortunately Carolyn's fragile health would again deteriorate and she passed away on Nov. 15th 2012.

Books & Resources that I found useful:

The Intelligent Patient Guide to Breast Cancer, Drs. Ivo Olivotto, Karen Gelmon, David McCready, Kathleen Pritchard, Urve Kuusk, (Intelligent Patient Guide Ltd. 2008)
Woman Cancer Sex, Anne Katz (Oncology Nursing Society Publishing Division, Hygeia Media, 2009)
Breast Cancer for Dummies
Intimacy After Cancer, Dr. Sally Kydd
The Breast Cancer Husband
Reconstructing Aphrodite, Dr. Loren Eskenazi, Dr. Susan Love, Terry Lorant, (Verve Editions, 2001)
Never Too Young
Life in the Balance
Getting Back on Track: Life after breast cancer treatment, Canadian Breast Cancer Foundation Ontario & Princess Margaret Hospital
The Healing Circle, Dr. Rob Rutledge, Timothy Walker, PhD. (Healing and Cancer Foundation, 2010)
Affirmations, Meditations and Encouragements for Women Living with Breast Cancer, Linda Dackman, (Harper Collins,1991)
Above and Beyond 365 Meditations for Transcending Chronic Pain and Illness, J.S. Dorian, (Plume Penguin, 1996)
Cancer Has Made Me a Shallower Person
Humor After the Tumor
Crazy Sexy Cancer

About the Author

Carolyn Schreuer was a devoted wife, mother, high-achiever and professional teacher in her mid-40s when she was diagnosed with breast cancer in 2009.

Before succumbing, she'd spend several years battling the disease, reassess her priorities, develop coping strategies and put all of her highly valuable insights and advice into her first and only book, *Carolyn & Cancer: Some Days I Don't Feel Like Slaying Dragons,* a helpful source of compassionate advice and a must-read for anyone facing serious illness.

Memorials

"Mom, this is exactly how I want to remember you... happy, strong, supportive, and beautiful! I love you! I hope you never forget me I promise I will never forget you."

- Daughter Victoria Schreuer

"August 21st, 1963-November 15th, 2012, a beautiful women lost her life to brain cancer. She was always smiling and the most happy person I have ever known. She fought so hard, from breast cancer, to bone cancer, to brain cancer she really did everything to fight this battle."

Son Wes

"I'm never going to forget your smile mom! Memories captured I will never forget. You were there for my very first breath, and I was there for your last. The time we got to share together, went by too quick... too fast."

- Daughter Victoria Schreuer

CAROLYN SCHREUER - August 21, 1963 - November 15, 2012 In Loving Memory of our Kind, Caring, Loving Daughter. Forever in our Hearts.
We love you.
Mom & Dad

"It is times like this I want to remember... its easy to remember sad and hard times because they are the most recent but I am glad that we had some happy times and I take comfort in knowing at one point we were happy and healthy now all I can hope for is that you are proud of me and who I am becoming... I know you are safe now but sometimes I wish I could hug you one more time."

- Daughter Victoria Schreuer

"One year ago today we said our final goodbye to one of the most beautiful people I have ever known. A woman who taught me so much about loving everyone, being as kind as you possibly can, embracing everything the world throws at you. I look at your beautiful children and know that you will live on in them. Your sense of humour in Wesley Snow, your love of children and your passion to teach and guide them in Victoria Schreuer, Carolyn Schreur, you will be missed by so many of us, forever. We will never forget you, your contagious smile, your way of finding the wonderful things in even the worst moment and your powerful fight. May you inspire us all every day. We love you."

Megg Scott Markettos

Carolyn Schreuer
Six months ago today our Caring, Sweet, Loving Daughter was
called to be with our Loving Saviour. We were all Blessed so
very much having you Carolyn. You were a Loving daughter,
sister, wife. mother and friend. You Loved so much and joyed in
helping others. You made this world a better place.
We Love You Carolyn.
(Jim Snow, dad, on May 15, 2013)

SCHREUER, Carolyn Marie (nee Snow) August 21, 1963 - November 15, 2012 Daughter, Sister, Wife, Mother, Teacher, Friend. After a long and courageous battle with cancer, Carolyn is finally at rest, but her legacy lives on. In her forty-nine years, Carolyn touched countless lives with her kindness, compassion, love and inspiration. Carolyn is survived by the love of her life, Wayne Schreuer, partner for over 30 years, husband for 23, and will be sadly missed by her two beautiful children Wesley and Victoria, the lights of her life. Carolyn is also survived by her parents Jim and Joanne Snow, her brothers Jeff Snow (Mary), Greg Snow (Claudine), her sister Marilyn Robichaud (Darren), also her nieces and nephews, Nick, Samantha, Katie, Emma, Ellie, Derek, Curtis and Alex. Beyond her family, Carolyn's love was extended to all her students. First as a teacher at Philip Pocock Catholic Secondary School in Mississauga and then at Sherwood Secondary School in Hamilton where she taught both English and her true calling, Cooperative Education. It is here that Carolyn influenced so many young people on their first steps into the working world. The support the Schreuer family has received throughout this journey has been overwhelming and we would like to thank everyone for their part in being one of our Angels watching over us. A special thank you to the staff on 3C JHCC and The Dr. Bob Kemp Hospice for their excellent care and kindness through the hardest days. Visitation will be held at DODSWORTH & BROWN Funeral Home, ANCASTER CHAPEL, 378 Wilson Street East, on Tuesday, November 20th from 5-9 p.m. and a Celebration of Life at the Beverly Golf Club on Wednesday, November 21st from 7-10 p.m. (1211 2nd Concession West, Copetown). Further, a Catholic mass and private family celebration will take place in the summer 2013, in Saint John, New Brunswick, Carolyn's first home. In lieu of flowers donations to the CIBC Breast Cancer Assessment Centre or Dr. Bob Kemp Hospice would be greatly appreciated.

Kindness can only be expected by the strong; it is the weak who are cruel. Go with the angels, my love, it is where you belong!

The family and friends of Carolyn

Manor House
905-648-2193